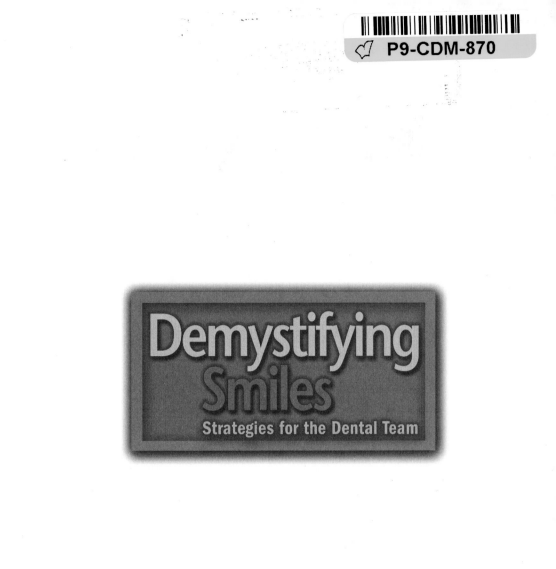

Demystifying Smiles
Strategies for the Dental Team

Demystifying Smiles:
Strategies for the Dental Team
By
Kristine A. Hodsdon, R.D.H., B.S.

With contributions from:

Bobbi Anthony, R.D.H.
Ann-Marie C. DePalma, R.D.H., B.S.
Deborah Dopson-Hartley, R.D.H.
Jeffery Dornbush, D.D.S.
Carol Jahn, R.D.H., M.B.A.
Jill Rethman, R.D.H., B.A.
Tricia Osuna, R.D.H., B.S.
Lynn D. Mortilla, R.D.H.
Donna M. Sirvydas, R.D.H., M.Ed.
Maria Perno Goldie, R.D.H., M.S.

Carol Jent, R.D.H., B.A.
Kathleen Johnson
Trish Jones, R.D.H., B.S.
Vicki McManus, R.D.H.
Mary Martineau, R.D.H.
Trisha E. O'Hehir, R.D.H., B.S.
Kristy Menage Bernie, R.D.H., B.S.
Karen Stueve, R.D.H.
Allison Roberts

PennWell®

Copyright© 2003 by
PennWell Corporation
1421 South Sheridan
Tulsa, Oklahoma 74112
800-752-9764
sales@pennwell.com
www.pennwell-store.com
www.pennwell.com

Cover designed by Amy Spehar
Book designed by Clark Bell

Library of Congress Cataloging-in-Publication Data

Hodsdon, Kristine A.
  Demystifying smiles : strategies for the dental team/by Kristine A. Hodsdon
       p. cm.
Includes bibliographical references and index.
  ISBN 0-87814-850-7
  1. Dentistry--Aesthetic aspects. Title.
  RK54 .H636 2002
  617.6--dc21
                                        2002038104

Printed in the United States of America

1 2 3 4 5   05 04 03 02 01

Table of Contents

Section I: Looking Through a Different Window

Section II: Hygiene Potential

SECTION III: TEAM ANTICS

List of Figures

Fig. 1–1: Fabricated IPS Empress restorations replacing the existing restorative dentistry, fabricated by Advanced Dental Technologies.

Fig. 1-2: Dental hygienist enrolling a patient for restorative care. (Courtesy of CAESY Education System)

Fig. 1–3: Maxillary occlusal view of the restorative dental condition prior to the 2001 treatment. There is evidence of tooth discoloration and fracture vulnerability from the existing amalgam restorations. The anterior four-unit fixed partial denture was fabricated in 1979, and there is a lingual collar display of gold from the supporting framework.

Fig. 1–4: The magnitude of the gold framework supporting the anterior fixed partial denture can be realized in this pretreatment 1999 radiographic series.

Fig. 1–5: At the time of the 2001 treatment, all existing restorative dentistry was taken out, the teeth were cleansed of decay, impressions made, and the provisional restoration was constructed using Zenith/DMG Luxatemp. Parameters for establishing occlusal relationships were worked out during the provisional phase of treatment.

Fig. 1–6: The stone cast with the definitive restorations fabricated by Jurium Dental Studio. The anterior fixed partial denture is a hybrid bridge consisting of feldspathic porcelain with a small embedded-cast framework.

Fig. 1–7: Occlusal view of the Targus Vectris posterior fixed partial denture restorations luted to place with Variolink II. Injection sites for the administration of the palatal technique to anesthetize maxillary anterior teeth are visible. The reduced bulk of the anterior feldspathic hybrid restoration is evident in the post-treatment full face and occlusal views.

Fig. 1–8: The post-treatment 2002 radiographic series illustrates the diminished bulk of the definitive restorations, which allows supra-gingival margin placement and creates an environment for periodontal health.

Fig. 1–9: A comparison of dental technology in 1978 and 2001 is demonstrated in these pre- and post-treatment photographs.

Fig. 2–1: Computerized checklists for a dental hygiene visit, courtesy of Pre-D Systems.

Fig. 2–2: The 3mm opening tip may be part of an aesthetic identification armamentarium (Surg-O-Vac courtesy of Young Dental).

Fig. 5–1: Cleaned and disinfected preparation, existing composite restoration, and occlusal grooves. Consepsis Scrub courtesy of Ultradent Products.

Fig. 5–2: A clean existing composite restoration, courtesy of Ultradent Products.

Fig. 5–3: Brush composite sealant vigorously into surface. PermaSeal, Courtesy of Ultradent Products.

Fig. 5–4: Four-year-old bonded Amelogen composite sealant, following a composite sealant treatment. PermaSeal, courtesy of Ultradent Products.

Fig. 5–5: Applying sealant. UltraSeal XT Plus, courtesy of Ultradent Products.

Fig. 5–6: Quality sealant. UltraSeal XT Plus, courtesy of Ultradent Products.

Fig. 6–1: Before and after photos of anterior sextant, dentistry courtesy of J. Schmid, D.D.S.; lab work by Aurum Ceramic.

Fig. 6–2: Before amalgam and after laboratory processes. Dentistry courtesy of Stephen Poss, D.D.S.; lab work by Aurum Ceramic.

Fig. 7–1: Example of an anterior color map, courtesy of the Las Vegas Institute of Advanced Dental Studies.

Fig. 7–2: Example of an anterior color map, courtesy of the Las Vegas Institute of Advanced Dental Studies.

Fig. 7–3: Example of a posterior color map, courtesy of the Las Vegas Institute of Advanced Dental Studies.

Acknowledgements

I could never have taken my professional journey, which has led to the writing of this manuscript, without the love and support of my best friend and husband, Mark J. Hodsdon. Mark and my children, Catherine and John, often heard

"In a minute," or

"Daddy will get that for you," or

"Everybody—please leave me alone!"

So, to them, *Demystifying Smiles* is dedicated.

The true heroes of this manuscript—the people who deserve special thanks and acknowledgment—are the contributors. They bestowed their spirit, passion, sense of humor, and willingness to give of themselves and their time to a collaborative manuscript. So I raise my proverbial beer bottle to them with a cheer:

Bobbi Anthony, R.D.H.; Ann-Marie C. DePalma, R.D.H., B.S.; Deborah Dopson-Hartley, R.D.H.; Jeffery Dornbush, D.D.S.; Carol Jahn, R.D.H., M.B.A.; Carol Jent, R.D.H., B.A.; Kathleen Johnson; Trish Jones, R.D.H., B.S.; Vicki McManus, R.D.H.; Mary Martineau, R.D.H.; Kristy Menage Bernie, R.D.H., B.S.; Lynn D. Mortilla, R.D.H.; Trisha E. O'Hehir, R.D.H., B.S.; Tricia Osuna, R.D.H., B.S.; Maria Perno Goldie, R.D.H., M.S.; Jill Rethman, R.D.H., B.A.; Allison Roberts; Donna M. Sirvydas, R.D.H., M.Ed.; Karen Stueve, R.D.H.

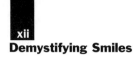

Foreword

by Michael Maroon, D.D.S. FAGD

Dentistry is an exciting and rewarding profession. How simple that statement is. Like any chosen career, dentistry will reward you for the amount of passion and enthusiasm that you bring to it.

One of the most exciting aspects of this profession has been the evolution of aesthetic materials and treatment over the last two decades. What is even more exciting is how patients have responded to this treatment. Many patients are changing the way that they view their visit to the dental office. Instead of the negativity that is often associated with a dental visit, there is a sense of gratitude. Patients are looking for ways to improve their appearance, health, and most importantly, the way they feel about themselves. More and more dental professionals are looking at the entire mouth and the importance of comprehensive dentistry when treating patients. Utilization of aesthetic materials has motivated many patients to treatment acceptance.

Dentistry today is ever more a "team" profession, and the successful treatment of the "aesthetic" patient is redefining the roles of each member of the team. From the first moment of contact with the office to the completion of treatment, it is important for everyone on the dental team to be "connected" and functioning together.

I am honored to write the foreword for this compilation, *Demystifying Smiles: Strategies for the Dental Team* because I know that you will enjoy learning from this group of esteemed professionals. Kristine A. Hodsdon, R.D.H., B.S., is an inspiration to anyone who has ever met her or read one of her published articles. She has evolved through all the changes that she is inviting you to discover. She has experienced the satisfaction that comes with treating patients successfully and being part of a dedicated team. She also understands the importance of passion and enthusiasm for your profession and has dedicated her professional life to sharing information and knowledge with others. She is a true leader and I am proud to be her friend.

In this book you will find examples, ideas, motivation, reasons, challenges, and more. It is a blueprint for success. Like any blueprint, it will remain on paper unless it is picked up by a builder and constructed into something beautiful.

My challenge to you is to take the information that is contained in this book and use it as a guideline to build your own vision of your practice. Live with passion. Be enthusiastic about what you do. You are changing lives. You are helping people to live longer. You are a dental professional. Congratulations!

Michael Maroon, D.D.S. FAGD

May 2002

Introduction

To laugh often and much; to win the respect of intelligent people and the affection of children; to earn the appreciation of honest critics and endure the betrayal of false friends; to appreciate beauty, to find the best in others; to leave the world a bit better, whether by a healthy child, a garden patch or a redeemed social condition; to know even one life has breathed easier because you have lived. This is the meaning of success. • **Ralph Waldo Emerson**

Congratulations! And welcome to a new world of increased awareness, the desire to deliver the best care, and the urge to make the most of your professionalism. By picking up this book, you have taken the first important step to move away from being a hygienist who only "scrapes teeth," a dental assistant who only "sucks spit," or an office manager who only "schedules appointments." I am not judging these career paths to be either good or bad. But if those are your only goals, then you may not hear the messages contained within this book. The audience for *Demystifying Smiles* is both the emerging and growing specialist and the knowledgeable professional who needs to be challenged and nudged to the next level.

Demystifying Smiles is unique. It is written for team members by team members: dental professionals who believe in the spirit of teams. My message is all about strategy sharing. My hope is that this book will speak to you.

First, a little background about myself. After graduating from hygiene school (my instructors deserve the hygiene Purple Heart!), painstakingly taking my clinical boards twice (another story), and finally receiving my license, I believed I had been ordained the evangelist of tooth brushing. My ministry was to rid the world of plaque, preaching from my ergonomically correct pulpit to one cleaning appointment at a time.

Later in my career, I was sort of born again, self-appointing myself the savior of aesthetic dental teams. My new mission was to single-handedly convert and open the eyes of dental teams everywhere to the power of aesthetics. Yes, overly ambitious, perhaps—but I realized that connecting with like-minded people makes magic!

With the opportunity to publish this book, write my columns and articles, and speak with audiences, I have been given a gift: To be able to retell others' triumphs and to share stories, plans, and ideas I have had the privilege to witness or hear about. My passion and knowledge rest squarely on the shoulders of enthusiasm from my audience members, the readers of my columns, my teachers and mentors, and even strangers who have contributed consciously or unconsciously their ideas and accomplishments. This book evolved and was inspired by my fortunate exposure to great and innovative minds that taught me and continue to teach me.

The ideas within these pages are not necessarily all new. More accurately, they will serve as a reminder of old ideas that somehow got lost or buried.

I organized this book into seven chapters. Each has a diverse array of topics, all in support of the general title of the chapter. The topics within each chapter are showcased in various avenues: Guest essays, "Kristineology", strategy tips, and action steps at the end of each chapter that will help you create your own professional game plan. I hope you will read the book cover to cover, but I realize that every practitioner may be seeking to customize his or her own reading/educational curriculum. In this spirit, each topic is indexed in the back.

Strategy Skill for Reading *Demystifying Smiles*

Step One: Identify a goal: What you want to accomplish.

Examples: Aesthetic enrollments

Clinical team management armamentarium

Finding self-product solutions

Providing complete care or business solutions

Step Two: Locate the section, chapter, or topic(s)

Step Three: Read it and lay out your action steps

Identify strategies and options

Step Four: Are there other ideas to consider?

Step Five: What support will you require?

Resources? Courses? Mentor?

Step Six: Outline your strategies in the back of the corresponding chapter

Step Seven: Detail or review your plan with the doctor and remaining team

Determine a date when you can begin your plan, how to chart progress, and areas where increased support is needed.

Add passion, brains, and competencies to the weave, and by working in collaboration as a team, everyone will be able to successfully integrate the strategies of the book.

Glossary of Terms

Some basic definitions will help clarify aesthetic and restorative options, which will provide team members with an enhanced ability to pre-diagnose the possibilities of the dental outcome and allow them to assist the dentist in differentiation diagnosis.

Take the opportunity to secure a mentoring relationship to determine "when each type of restoration is indicated," and/or any alternative treatments. Create (or purchase) practice-centered marketing materials, post-treatment written instructions, and practice your presentation skills.

Air Abrasion. Air abrasion is a technique that can be used to prepare different types of cavity preparations, some restoration repair, and sandblasting procedures.

Block-Out Resins. Block-out resins are light-cured resins that can be used as a rubber dam substitute when fabricating whitening trays; as a protection intraorally during sandblasting; to block out imperfections during final impressions; and as an added protection during power whitening.

Caries Detecting Dyes. Caries detecting dyes are used to assist the clinician in determining between affected and infected dentin.

Cavity Cleaners/Disinfectants. Cavity cleaners/disinfectants can be used during adhesion procedures (such as sealant application or indirect bonding), as well as removing any left over provisional cement.

Ceramics. Ceramic materials are tooth-colored, glass-like, porcelain-based fillings. They are fabricated in a laboratory (indirect restoration) and can be used for both anterior and posterior teeth. Ceramic material can be used in ceramomental and all-ceramic restorations (crowns, inlays, veneers, etc.).

Compomer. Compomers are polyacid-modified composite that can release fluoride.

Composite. Composites are tooth-colored, plastic-based materials that can be used as anterior or posterior restorations.

Composite Reinforcement Fibers. Composite reinforcement fibers are materials that can increase flexural strength of restorations, bridges, posts, cores, etc., as well as periodontal splints and orthodontic retainers.

Composite Sealants. Composite sealants are unfilled resins that are designed to fill in the microcracks and or microscopic defects after an adhesion or finishing procedure.

Dental Adhesion. Dental adhesion includes systems and techniques that allow a dentist to adhere dental materials to natural tooth structures.

Desensitizers. Desensitizers are used to minimize or eliminate sensitive areas and teeth. The product category includes toothpaste, fluorides, gels, and varnishes.

Direct Restoration (direct bonding). An anterior or posterior restoration that can be placed in one appointment.

Hybrid. Hybrids are part of the composite family. As restorations, they are known for their strength and polishability.

Implants. Dental Implants are components that can be placed in the upper or lower jawbone. These devices, once placed, can be used to support crowns, bridges, and other restorative dentistry.

Indirect Resin Systems. Indirect resin systems are laboratory-fabricated restorations that share the advantages of being part of the composite resin category. Their indications may be anterior veneers and or posterior restorations.

Indirect Restoration (indirect bonding): After the dentist preps a tooth or teeth, an impression is taken and sent to a laboratory. The dental laboratory, in partnership with the dentist, fabricates the restoration on a stone model made from the impression.

Magnification Systems. Magnification systems are units that increase a clinician's ability to see in the oral environment. They are must-have instruments for *all* clinical doctors and team members

Microfill. Microfills are part of the composite resin family. As restorations, they are known for their ability to mirror enamel and polishability to a high shine.

Radiometers (light meters). Light meters allow a clinician to check the effectiveness of a curing light.

Resin Cements. Resin cements are modified composites that are used to bond indirect restorations.

Restorative Polishing Pastes. Polishing pastes, either for composite or ceramic restorations, have the ability to add a "luster" to a newly placed restoration and/or remove stain during hygiene management sessions.

Rubber Polishing Instruments. Rubber polishing instruments are used to polish and renew composites and or ceramic restorations.

Sealants. Sealants are modified composites that are placed in the pit and fissure of the occlusal surface of teeth.

Masticatory System Related Terms

Understanding some basic concepts will allow team members to recognize the trust value of complete aesthetic and restorative dentistry as it relates to optimum health. These definitions are a starting point for team members who have had little exposure to these concepts. This list is based on terms I have collected and found useful in my ongoing enlightenment about occlusion.

Since there is no holy grail of occlusion, get in the game by developing a mentoring relationship with someone who can support your learning efforts.

Anterior Digastric Muscle. A main muscle involved in jaw opening.

Anterior Guidance. Think of it as the front leg of an upside-down, three-legged stool. The rear legs of the stool can symbolize the right and left temporo-mandibular units. Anterior guidance is the most anterior factor or contact and the first occlusal contact to occur on one or more teeth when closing the mandible against the maxillary. It is believed that the anterior (or front, healthy teeth) are best suited for this initial contact, to carry the load or simultaneous contacts.

Canine Guidance. Similar to the incisal guidance theory, but the overbite and overjet relationship is applied to the canines.

Centric Relation: Closing of the jaws in a position that provides maximum contact between the occluding surfaces of the maxillary and mandibular arch. It may be achieved through mechanical or bilateral manipulation.

Incisal Guidance. The movement of the lingual surfaces of the maxillary incisors and the incisal edges of the mandibular incisors, such as the overbite-overjet relationship.

Lateral Excursion. The mandible travels from the resting position to the right or left until cuspids on that side are in cusp to the cusp position. In that position, the teeth on the other side should not be in contact.

Lateral Pterygoid Muscle. A main muscle involved in jaw opening.

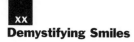

Laterotrusive Movement. Mandible moves to the right or left.

Load Testing. Used for verification of complete condylar seating in centric relation.

Masseter Muscle. A muscle that is involved in jaw closing.

Maximal Intercuspal Position. Maximum intercuspal positions or inter-cuspal position is a definite and stable end point of closure. Synonyms may include maximal occlusal contact position or vertical dimension.

Maximum Incisal Opening (MIO). Measured from the incisal edges of the center incisors when the mandible is opened to its furthest extent.

Medial Pterygoid Muscle. This muscle is involved in jaw closing.

Midline Shift. The midline of the central incisors shift either left or right.

Muscles of Mastication. Masseter, temporal, medial pterygoid muscle, lateral pterygoid, and digastric.

Myo-Centric/Neuromuscular. A physiologic stable jaw-joint position that is achieved with the least amount of muscle energy and accommodation to bring the mandible into intercuspation. This position is achieved by electrical stimulation (TENS) of relaxed masticatory muscles.

Neutral Zone/Neutral Space. The space that houses the lip-teeth-tongue. Balance is attained when the eruptional forces of the teeth, the out-ward forces of the tongue (strength of the tongue), and the inner force of the lips (tightness of the lip, lower lip), are all in harmony with one another. Tongue thrust is an example of a disturbance of the neutral zone.

Nonsupporting Cusps. The buccal cusps of the maxillary teeth and the lin-gual cusps of the mandibular teeth, which do not generally support vertical dimension.

Non-Working (balancing side). Posterior teeth should disclude without interferences.

Occlusal Relationship. The marriage of the lower teeth to the upper teeth.

Open Bite. The lack of occlusion of maxillary and mandibular arches.

Overbite. The vertical overlap of the maxillary incisors against the corre-sponding mandible incisors.

Overjet. The horizontal overlap of the maxillary incisors against the corre-sponding mandibular incisors.

Pathway/Arc of Opening or Closing. The straight or linear path of opening and closing of the mandible.

Periodontal Ligament. The band of soft connective tissue that connects the tooth root to the alveolar bone.

Posterior Guidance. Similar to the anterior overjet-overbite relationship, but now applied to the posterior regions during lateral extrusion movements.

Premature Contact/Interference. If, during closing or mandibular movement, a tooth (teeth) prevents the anterior teeth to contact first and may interfere with the condlye position. For example, this interference may be a high restoration that prevents the front teeth from contacting first. Synonyms may include anterior support, anterior determinant, and anterior control.

Protrusive Movement. Mandibular movement forward from the intercuspal position. During normal mandibular protrusive movement, the anterior teeth should shoulder the contacts and the posterior teeth should disclude without interferences.

Supporting Cusps. The cusps of the maxillary and mandibular teeth that support the vertical dimension or provide the most stable copal position.

Temporalis Muscle. A muscle that is involved in jaw closing.

Transcutaneous Electrical Nerve Stimulation (TENS). TENS delivers a low frequency, low-voltage neuromuscular stimulation to the identified masticatory muscles, for the purpose of relaxation.

Vertical Dimension. Vertical dimension can be described as the vertical facial height or distance between the arches. It is achieved by the relationship of the supporting/centric cusps of the maxillary and mandibular teeth.

Working Side. Posterior teeth should disclose and work in harmony with the anterior guidance.

Light Curing

Quartz Tungsten Halogen (QTH). QTH bulbs use a heated tungsten filament to release radiation. Only 0.5% of the radiation is useful for light curing, the remaining is heat. These sources need adequate cooling.

Plasma Arc Curing (PAC). PAC lights are short-arc xenon bulbs that use tungsten electrodes in a xenon gas environment. The electrical arc ionizes that gas at a high temperature, producing plasma that produces very high radiation output.

Laser. Argon ion lasers emit a blue-green high-energy beam from energized argon atoms. The wavelengths are usually well matched with composite resin initiators, such as CQ with little heat.

LED. Light-emitting diodes. An emerging technology in light-curving units.

Champhorquinone (CQ). CQ is one composite initiator in dental resins that is cured by a light source. In earlier generations of composite development, CQ was the stand-alone initiator, manufactured to be cured with a halogen-type light. With the plethora of material composition available today, and with developments in light technology, it is imperative to make sure you have a lock-and-key scenario. That is: the composite photopolymerization process (curing process ingredients) can be initiated by the light source being utilized.

mW/cm2. milliWatt [mW] per centimeter squared [cm2]

Continuous Cure. In a continuous cure mode, a light source emitting constant intensity is applied to a composite for a specific period of time. This is the most universal method of curing.

Stepped Cure. In a stepped cure mode, a composite is first cured at low energy and then stepped up to a higher energy, each for a set time frame.

Ramp Cure. In this case, light is initially applied at low intensity and gradually increased over time to high intensity.

High Energy Pulse Cure. This technique uses a very brief pulse of extremely high energy, which is three- to six-times the normal power dentistry.

Pulse Delay Cure. In this discontinuous mode, a single pulse of light is applied to a restoration, followed by a second pulse, and then by a third-pulse cure of greater intensity and longer duration, in an interrupted step increase.

Building Blocks of Color

When light passes through tooth structure, it can be reflected, refracted, absorbed, or transmitted by all the layers of a tooth. This varying optical distinctiveness gives the natural tooth a multicolor or polychromatic effect.

Chroma. Chroma may be defined as the strength or purity of the hue. The term saturation is frequently used instead of chroma and the two are largely interchangeable. Other synonyms are intensity and concentration. Pale colors and pastels are of low chroma; intense, strongly hued colors have a high chroma. To use an analogy, imagine a glass of red wine. Now add water to the wine. The chromatic part of the wine will decrease in intensity as more water is added, but the hue remains the same.

Fluorescence. When ultraviolet (UV) lights are absorbed by the enamel and dentin and emit a brilliance that can enhance the brightness or value of the tooth (teeth.)

Hue. Hue is the attribute of color or shade (red, blue, or yellow) that is most frequently confused with color itself. Remember, hue is one of the *three* dimensions of color.

Opalescence. Iridescent appearance when a surface is illuminated by light.

Translucency and Opacity. These degrees are determined by the tooth structure (enamel and dentin) and thickness and the amount of light that passes through them.

Value. Value is the relative blackness or whiteness of a color. On a scale of black to white, white is a high value, black, a low value, with median gray midway between black and white. Value is the only dimension of color that may exist by itself. A black-and-white photograph is a *one-dimensional* rendition of a three-dimensional object. Additionally, some clinicians determine the value of a color by comparing black-and-white photographs of teeth with a guide featured in the picture.

Basic Research Terminology

Bond Strength. Adhesion strength of the cement or bonding agent

Crossover. Different subjects are compared to one another at one point in time.

Double-Blind Study. Neither the subjects nor the investigator/researcher know whom the control or treatment group is.

Efficacy. The degree to which a treatment is beneficial when implemented under the usual conditions of an investigation, usually a randomized clinical trial.

Evidence-Based Care. The conscientious and judicious use of current best evidence from clinical care research in the management of individual patients.

Hawthorne Effect. A subject (P) will perform better because he or she is in a study. If P is greater than .05, it is not statistically significant (P>.05); if P is less than .05, it is statistically significant (P<. 05).

In vitro. Studies done within an artificial or laboratory environment.

In vivo. Studies done within a living organism on human subjects.

Mean. The sum of all the observations divided by the number of observation.

Median. A measure of central location.

Mode. Most frequently occurring value among all the observations in a sample.

N=. Specific number of subjects who are included in a study.

Randomized Clinical Trial. A study in which a group receiving an experimental treatment is compared with a control receiving a placebo or standard treatment.

SEM. Scanning electron microscopy

Single-Blind Study. The investigator/researcher does not know which group of subjects are the control or the treatment group.

Standard Deviation. A measure of dispersion in the way a list of numbers spreads out around its average.

Statistically Significant. A meaningful or important result observed from one therapy compared with another therapy.

Tensile Load. Pulling tension placed on a bonded restoration to the point that it is affected.

Section I

Looking Through A Different Window

ONE
Understanding the Bigger Picture

The farther backward you look, the farther forward you are likely to see. • **Winston Churchill**

Show Up, Connect, and Infect

My observation is that many team members are not clear on what they want for themselves professionally and do not actually know what business their practices are in. Getting a plan established that consistently provides comprehensive restorative, aesthetic, and periodontal care takes a true team. It takes a shared vision, and it takes independent knowledge.

Success means many different things to many people. Our vision of success is usually measured by our own set of values and goals. Our individual values and goals make up our personal and professional vision.

So, it is discouraging for me to hear that a team member feels pressure to "sell" cosmetic services, or is having some personal conflicts with the office demands. Rallying the practice troops to take sides, or attempting to undermine the doctor/owner, will not solve anything. You, as an individual, must discover what business you are in. Some or all of the following questions may help to clarify your own professional mission. There are no right or wrong answers—only those answers that fit your professional principles.

Ask yourself:

- How do I want to help others? Why?
- What will make me happy in my work? Why?
- What is my standard of care? And why?
- What type of environment do I choose to work in? Why?
- What is my goal when serving my patients?
- What are my beliefs about comprehensive periodontal, aesthetic, and restorative dentistry?
- What is my ideal smile?
- How do I feel about having optimal aesthetic and restorative dentistry in my mouth?
- What am I willing to do, change, or risk to practice within a team?
- What are the professional goals that I want to achieve?
- How will I go about designing my own professional growth curriculum?

If you cannot answer these introspective questions or visualize your ideal practice environment, or finish statements like "I will be happy professionally when . . . ," how are you able to deliver care in the environment in which you are currently working? Or, if you already know you are unhappy in your current work situation and want to make a shift to a new dental employment home, how will you know what to look for the next time, without clarifying what you want? Or—equally as powerful—what you do not want?

Because the "practice" of dental hygiene is actually a "practice within a practice," and because dental assistants usually work interdependently with the doctor, it is imperative that all team members and the doctor share not only values and goals, but also a vision of where they want to take the practice. This aligned vision is like a road map to the practice they wish to create.

How can everyone be expected to reach the same destination if they don't share the same map? If the doctor is heading down one road and a certain team member is driving in another direction, neither will have created what they wished for—and both will feel dissatisfied, frustrated, and possibly even under-appreciated or burned out. An impasse to success in many dental practices is this difference between the doctor's paradigm of success and that of the team's.

Though all parties may share the values of high quality care and concern for patients, for example, the players may have very different visions of what those values may look like in a practice.

For instance, what if the hygienist's vision of "concern for the patient" includes worrying about what the patient can afford, or he or she believes that cosmetic dentistry is optional dentistry that only a particular segment of the patient base can afford? The dentist, in fact, may feel very differently about those values. The dentist may feel that patients should have the right to choose for themselves whatever level of care they feel is appropriate. The reality falls somewhere in the middle, but this difference of vision could create aggravation between the doctor and the hygienist and create dissatisfaction for the entire team. However, if the vision for the practice has been fully articulated by the doctor and all aspects of the goals and values discussed, then the collaboration among doctor and team may have the opportunity to grow into an ownership-shared vision.

Ownership is a powerful tool that can move people much more quickly toward the realization of their goals. This partnership and vision can ensure that all parties are traveling the same road in the same direction at the same speed.

Now, it is time to make clear the distinctions of your current practice. Ask yourself the following:

What is the mission of my practice?

- Is my professional mission congruent with my current work atmosphere?
- Do I own that vision and mission with the doctor and the rest of the team?
- What knowledge will I have to gain to support that shared vision?
- What services does the practice want to provide—smile enhancement, periodontal, total-health, emergent care, orthodontics, etc.?
- Do I believe in all the services my office provides?

- What services may need to be reconsidered or added in order to support the shared vision?
- What are the elective services that I am uncomfortable with recommending, and why?
- What are my concerns and questions about these services?
- And finally, do I need to make some dramatic changes in my attitude, beliefs, and behaviors?

This self-actualization and practice analysis will better prepare you for a genuine discussion with your employer and other team members.

If you feel that your fellow team members are traveling down different roads—if your office is not working together cohesively—speak up! Ask to schedule a team meeting. Start the meeting by explaining your desire to understand the doctor's vision for the practice, to learn what other team members are looking for, and to establish a clear set of expectations for all.

Then, do some soul searching to determine your role and how you see yourself functioning in the practice. Clarify your expectations so that they mesh with an office mission or philosophy that is a healthier way to practice. Discovering what business your practice is in, clarifying what services you provide, determining what best serves the people whom you treat—and making sure all are harmonious—will help disarm negative judgments that patients make about a dysfunctional team.

Example of an Aesthetic Team Mission. Delivering clinical, behavioral, administrative, and personal services within the comprehensive framework of the theories and best practices of aesthetic dentistry. (Fig. 1–1)

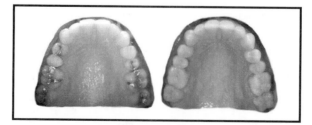

Fig. 1–1: *Fabricated IPS Empress restorations replacing the existing restorative dentistry, fabricated by Advanced Dental Technologies.*

Did We Expect to Learn It All in School?

by Jeffery Dornbush, D.D.S.

I graduated from the New York University College of Dentistry in February 1975 after only three-and-a-half years of formal dental education. We were the transitional class, as the dental school attempted to pare its four-year curriculum to three years. There was much controversy about whether we were adequately prepared for our clinical careers in just three- and-a-half years. It seemed as if the goal of our dental educators was to teach all that we had to know by graduation. Despite my continued pursuit of knowledge in the postgraduate prosthodontics program at Boston University School of Graduate Dentistry, the notion that a formal dental education would prepare us to cope with everything we need to know was dispelled early on.

Looking back with the wisdom of 20-20 hindsight, the metamorphosis that has occurred within what is considered "known" in nearly every discipline of dentistry has been substantial. I can see why this quote is apropos.

It is what you learn after you think you know it all that counts.
• **John Wooden**

In many instances, the way we practice dentistry today is the opposite of the way I was taught to practice in 1975. For example, consider the difference between the fundamentals in 1975 and in 2002.

Participation over many years in hundreds of hours of continuing education, from both the student and teaching perspective, calls for acknowledgement of available postgraduate educational opportunities. Without the ongoing efforts of those active within these institutions, we would not be where we are today.

The process of implementing advances to our clinical practice demands our learning and continuing education, although it can be steeped in controversy. The German philosopher Arthur Schopenhauser said:

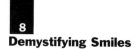

All truth goes though three steps.
First, it is ridiculed.
Second, it is violently opposed.
Finally, it is accepted as self-evident.

For example, during the process of incorporating any of the following procedures, we may be chided as being a "bond-o-dontist," a "white-tooth specialist," a "techie," or a cosmetic dentist who gives everyone implants, bleaching, or veneers.

Today's vast advances in media technology mean people are more knowledgeable about what will be going on in their mouths. In 1975, patients were usually informed of indications for treatment to alleviate common complaints of pain and tooth loss, but there existed a shroud of mystery about what dentistry was actually doing for them. Now, patients often come in and ask for treatment! Our ready-at-hand tools for interactive education and effective communication between doctor and patient make our jobs easier. Increased patient/doctor understanding demystifies the whole process. There is less anxiety and this also facilitates better communication. For example, our dental operatory may be equipped with 20-inch video monitors for patient viewing of intraoral images and interactive patient-education programs, such as CAESY DVD formats and instructional videotapes. In addition, a separate computer monitor placed discretely behind the patient in the operatory allows access to practice management software (such as Dentrix Multi-User Software), digital camera images, and cosmetic imaging software (such as Image F/X). (Fig. 1-2)

In fact, the entire realm of audio, video, and computer technology facilitates the manner in which we make case presentations to our patients. Another valuable resource is photographs (or 35-mm slides) of previously treated cases, which are readily accessible for viewing by a prospective patient. Photographs and slides can conveniently be organized and stored as a digital library. Scanned into a digital format, they may be put into categories such as periodontal, prosthesis, crown-and-bridge, implant-supported restorations, aesthetic porcelain-laminate veneers, and amalgam replacement, with all-ceramic restorative dentistry. Storage for this digital library of case-presentation material is conveniently achieved by creating a CD-ROM using a CD burner. A CD-ROM containing before-and-after photos for illustrating clinical scenarios is easily accessed from any computer. In addition to case presentations, the digital format is conveniently available for web site development and patient education.

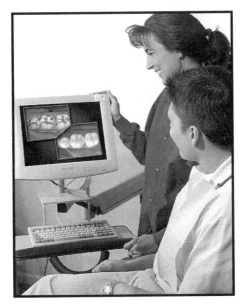

Fig. 1-2: *Dental hygienist enrolling a patient for restorative care.*
(Courtesy of CAESY Education System)

The following documentation of treatment provided for my wife exemplifies a comparison of trends in dental care available in 1975 with those of today. (Figs. 1–3 through 1–9) The "yellow" character of her dentition prior to the advent of tooth whitening dictated the chroma of her four-unit, upper anterior, fixed partial denture that was fabricated for her in 1979. The two central incisors are pontics supported by the lateral incisor abutments. In the retracted pretreatment photo, a luting agent washout of the retainer of the upper right lateral incisor (#7) is evidenced by redness of the marginal gingival tissue.

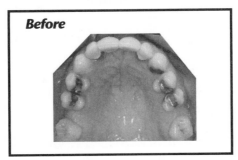

Fig. 1–3: *Maxillary occlusal view of the restorative dental condition prior to the 2001 treatment. There is evidence of tooth discoloration and fracture vulnerability from the existing amalgam restorations. The anterior four-unit fixed partial denture was fabricated in 1979, and there is a lingual collar display of gold from the supporting framework.*

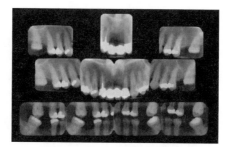

Fig. 1–4: *The magnitude of the gold framework supporting the anterior fixed partial denture can be realized in this pretreatment 1999 radiographic series.*

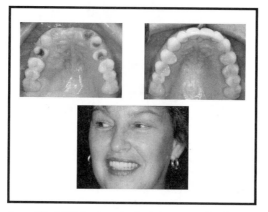

Fig. 1–5: *At the time of the 2001 treatment, all existing restorative dentistry was taken out, the teeth were cleansed of decay, impressions made, and the provisional restoration was constructed using Zenith/DMG Luxatemp. Parameters for establishing occlusal relationships were worked out during the provisional phase of treatment.*

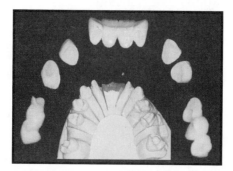

Fig. 1–6: *The stone cast with the definitive restorations fabricated by Jurium Dental Studio. The anterior fixed partial denture is a hybrid bridge consisting of feldspathic porcelain with a small embedded-cast framework.*

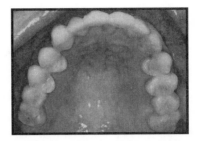

Fig. 1-7: *Occlusal view of the Targus Vectris posterior fixed partial denture restorations luted to place with Variolink II. Injection sites for the administration of the palatal technique to anesthetize maxillary anterior teeth are visible. The reduced bulk of the anterior feldspathic hybrid restoration is evident in the post-treatment full face and occlusal views.*

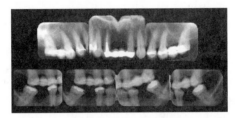

Fig. 1-8: *The post-treatment 2002 radiographic series illustrates the diminished bulk of the definitive restorations, which allows supra-gingival margin placement and creates an environment for periodontal health.*

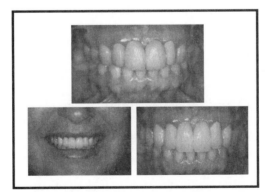

Fig. 1-9: *A comparison of dental technology in 1978 and 2001 is demonstrated in these pre- and post-treatment photographs.*

At times, it may seem overwhelming to learn and implement the vast array of advances pertinent to our clinical practices. It has been helpful to keep in mind a quotation by Henry Ford: "Nothing is particularly hard if you divide it into small jobs."

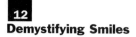

Merging of the Occlusion

Have you ever wondered why one tooth-colored material appears durable and remains aesthetically pleasing in a patient's mouth, while the same material fractures or breaks down in another's? Or, when evaluating current conditions in a patient's mouth, have you ever noticed an excessive amount of broken posterior teeth or restorations, tooth sensitivity, localized periodontal concerns, and/or muscle problems? Have you ever noted occlusal interferences during opening, closing, lateral, or protrusive movements? Clinical findings in these and other areas may indicate occlusal management problems.

Dental hygienists and clinical assistants are not trained in school to recognize and understand the detailed connection between teeth and the muscles that support the head, neck, jaw joints, face, etc. Those who take the initiative to learn about these connections—through continuing education and by learning advanced occlusion principles—and then apply that knowledge during pre-diagnostic examinations will improve their contribution to the clinical success and longevity of restorative/aesthetic and cosmetic dentistry.

For instance: Have you witnessed clinical failures with some of the modern materials? It may not be faulty restorative product properties, but rather, inappropriate case selection and a lack of focus on comprehensive treatment planning to include the occlusal scheme and muscle forces. For example, if a patient exhibits a pathologic occlusion prior to treatment, and the condition is undiagnosed or not treated, the occlusal force will either destroy the restorative material and/or the opposing dentition, or cause the patient post-operative tooth or jaw pain—no matter what restorative material is used. For a restorative material to survive in the mouth, clinicians must control as many biomechanical force loads as possible.

So, to re-emphasize: If hygienists and dentists are not taking the time to provide a complete occlusal evaluation, they should not be surprised or frustrated when tooth-colored restorations fracture or show signs of wear, or when they hear post-operative complaints about tooth sensitivity or jaw aches.

Understanding the essentials of occlusal and functional concepts supports true comprehensive care and a total oral wellness plan. Gaining such insights helps to break the cycle of ambiguous crown or amalgam placement, which leads to destructive consequences, such as fractured restorations or increased occlusal pathology. Being mentored about the intricacies of occlusion, the diagnostic aids, and the steps for treatment involves a congruency among the entire staff, but it can set the practice apart from others, by providing full-mouth care in the community.

Reading the "signs and symptoms"

Hygienists and team members understand that aesthetics is more than cosmetics and a practice's vision for providing comprehensive dentistry. But they should understand the multiple factors of occlusion in relation to comprehensive care, and be able to identify clinical signs and symptoms during clinical sessions.

Hygienists, specifically, are the team members with the most consistent access to the patient base through recare. A registered dental hygienist's knowledge of the functional reasons for aesthetic dentistry is imperative. Otherwise, many full-mouth cases could walk out the door undiagnosed.

Below are examples of questions to consider during hygiene screening.

1. Do you have, or have you ever had problems with your jaw, or had any injury to your jaw or face area?
2. Are you aware of, or ever had any pain/discomfort when you chew, talk, "open too wide," or close?
3. Do you hear or have ever heard grating, clicks, pops?
4. Does your jaw ever stick, lock, or has it ever "gone out"?
5. Do you or have you ever had difficulty chewing or eating?
6. Are you aware of any grinding or clenching of your teeth?
7. Have you noticed your teeth getting shorter, longer, or chipping easily?

Since occlusal discrepancies can be multi-factoral, no one cause-and-effect relationship can be easily isolated. Clinical signs to consider include the following:

- Class V non-carious lesions
- Para-functional habits (clenching; grinding; biting on pens, pins, or nails; unusual postural habits, etc.)
- Protrusive movements (mandible moves forward)
- Heavy lateral forces (mandible moves from left to right across the maxillary arch)
- Premature occlusal contacts, uncoordinated muscle function
- Tooth mobility
- Open contacts
- Titling or drifting of teeth
- Changes in percussive sounds
- Extreme occlusal wear
- Changes in radiographic anatomy (site-specific variations of the lamina dura, variations of the periodontal space, root fractures, root resorption, hypercementosis, and/or pulpal calcifications)
- Localized soft tissue changes

If a patient answers "yes" to any of the screening questions and/or during the hygiene screening, or if any of the clinical signs are recorded, a hygienist should inform and educate the patient that there may be a concern with how his/her teeth align with each other.

Until recently, the diagnostic tools that clinicians had, such as articulating paper, were not always sensitive enough to determine what was wrong with a patient's bite. In the mid-1990s, an emerging technology called T-Scan (Tekscan, www.tekscan.com) began to aid in the clinician's ability to accurately develop a well-balanced occlusal treatment plan. When a patient bites on a sensor, data are fed into a software program located on a laptop or conventional computer. The T-scan then uses vivid graphics to show results that can be viewed by the clinician and patient. This technology also includes a video component that allows hygienists to measure and see the sequential relationship/forces of the bite.

For comparison, articulating paper can only measure where the patient is biting, i.e., the contact points. T-scan monitors the strength of the force of closure and pressure on each tooth. This information gives clinicians the ability to determine if the patient's teeth are hitting evenly upon closure, or if there is a premature contact of one tooth or a few teeth that interferes with the closure pattern, and thus interfering with all teeth contacting appropriately and so preventing full intercuspation. (Maximum intercuspal position is a definite and stable end point of jaw closure.) This is an invaluable technology for a hygiene department that is easily incorporated into the hygiene assessment phase of service. The evaluation can be performed and the results displayed on the screen and completed in a timely sequence prior to the doctor's examination.

The doctor, upon reviewing the assessment findings, provides a more complete examination and differential diagnosis of the variation and/or provides necessary therapeutic choices.

Hygiene occlusal analysis steps

- Observe and record standards and deviations (T-bite)
- Angle's classification
  - Normal occlusion
  - Class I malocclusion
  - Class II malocclusion
  - Class III malocclusion
- Overbite/ overJet/ open bite
- Maximal incisal opening (MIO)
- Arc of closure
- Occlusal interferences
- Discrepancies in protrusive/ lateral movements

Team members and doctors need to take the opportunity to discuss, develop, and implement protocols, skills, understandings, and rationale to support form-and-function communication and the coordination of re-enrolling patients of record for comprehensive examination of care.

Smile! You're on a Dental Camera!

Whether or not you provide smile-enhancement dentistry or a hygiene service, make sure that you have a complete photography survey completed. It's fun and will allow you to walk in the patient's shoes. Photography strategies—whether taking or assisting—include the following tips:

- Keep the mirror dry (moist-free)
- Rest mirror on opposing arch
- Try to see the facial or anterior teeth
- Remember to include first molars

Curing light strategy

A curing light's baseline intensity should be measured with a radiometer when a curing light is new and, subsequently, at least weekly.

When curing a composite, sealant, or whitening—when utilizing any power light source—follow the manufacturer's instructions as to duration and distance. It is imperative that we do not "doze off" when using a curing light, because excessive heat, possible pulpal damage, and/or lip, tongue, or gingival burning may result.

Restorations and/or sealants cured with inadequate light intensity can result in sensitivity, breakdown, failure, unhappy patients, and, ultimately, loss of income due to the time needed for replacement of dentistry—and patients!

Barrier protection can be used with curing light tips, but they may decrease or interfere with the light-output intensity. Test the light output with a commercial radiometer, with and without barrier protection (even a Mylar strip), and record any difference. Then adjust curing time accordingly.

Keep curing tips free of debris and old resin, which may decrease the lights' effectiveness.

Always turn off a curing unit once the fan has stopped running. If turned off while the fan is still running, the unit could overheat.

Create Your Strategies

If you are not ready today, you will be even less ready tomorrow. •
Ovid

This exercise is provided at the end of each chapter to assist you in designing a game plan based on each chapter's topics. It will help you develop the skills, knowledge, and expertise necessary to propel you to your next level of personal and professional growth. Ask, answer, and record the following:

My professional goals for understanding comprehensive care in the future are:

_____

_____

_____

The areas for which I would like assistance and support to achieve my goals are:

_____

_____

_____

My action steps to get in the game and achieve those goals are:

_____

_____

_____

My list of specific goals and dates I wish to accomplish them includes:

_____

_____

_____

Possible obstacles to watch out for: (i.e., fear of rejection, fear of change, lack of accountability, denial, lack of focus, lack of self-evaluation, lack of mentoring relationships):

_____

_____

_____

TWO

Team Possible:
Becoming Aesthetic Detectives

Genius is the ability to reduce the complicated to the simple.
• CW Ceran

Aesthetic Attitude

The connection between comprehensive care and aesthetic dentistry is alive and unshakable. When a dental practice is shifting its focus from traditional restorative services to providing more comprehensive smile design modalities, it is up to the team to make their office survive and thrive!

All team members must be enthusiastic and well versed in discussing aesthetic materials and procedures. The hygiene relationship of two, three, four, and/or six-month intervals, for example, can give patients an intimate, secure, and non-threatening environment in which to share what they want to achieve with their overall oral health.

Second, hygiene sessions allow for the patient's subjective smile needs and wants to be discovered, rediscovered, and recorded during the smile evaluation and assessment phases of the dental hygiene process of care. This in turn provides an ongoing opportunity for the hygienist to educate the patient to understand his or her aesthetic options. These steps can be executed while positioning the dental hygienist as a professional team player and an advocate of aesthetic treatments. (Fig. 2-1)

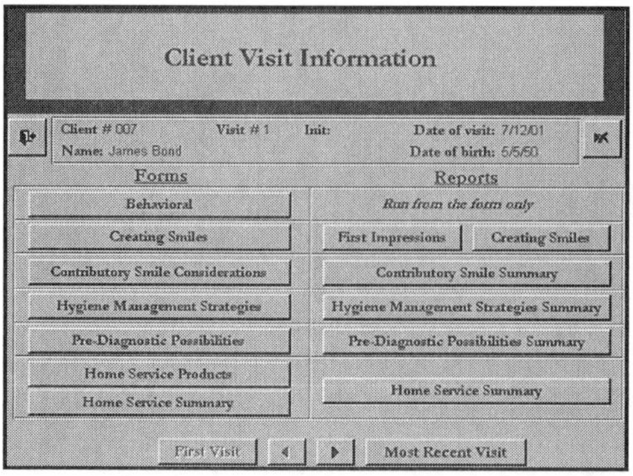

Fig. 2–1: *Computerized checklists for a dental hygiene visit, courtesy of Pre-D Systems.*

Team members must be not just *knowledgeable* about the procedures of restorative and aesthetic dentistry, but *passionate*. The passion must come from designing integrated hygiene and restorative departments that support the practice's restorative and smile design vision.

The first step in establishing and maintaining an aesthetic and cosmetic focus is attitude! Before anything else, a certified dental assistant must believe that the alternatives to amalgam, porcelain-fused-to-metal, and smile design principles are research-validated services and superior restorative options. Patient appointment coordinators must understand that amalgams and metal restorations are not unhealthy, but that newer materials and adhesive (bonding) methods, when performed with precision and excellence, allow for lifelike appearance and clinical reliability. The techniques allow the restoring dentist to *add* materials to a tooth instead of constantly *subtracting* tooth structure in order to build up or restore the tooth.

Numerous restorative systems are available, and a team member must understand that composite and ceramic restorations are well-accepted treatment modalities. Generally, clinical and retrospective studies document that bonded ceramic and composite materials show successful clinical versatility and longevity—anywhere from 5 to 12 (or more) years.

These modern treatment alternatives are valuable tools for restoring teeth, but they require a significant amount of pre-diagnostic and diagnostic information-gathering and clinical skills. Continuing education, to expand one's thinking and clinical abilities, is a basic component that must be considered when transforming a practice into a comprehensive aesthetic model. Comprehensive dental- and hygiene-care plans for long-term stability must begin with perfect periodontal tissue and continue restoratively with what is biologically acceptable, functionally long lasting, and aesthetically pleasing.

The second part of the aesthetic frame of mind occurs when the team learns and exhibits constant support and belief in the abilities of the clinical dentist. This faith must not be as a blind, ignorant, cult-like following! As licensed and certified professionals who provide care to the public, our heads and hearts must be in alignment with our team's and with our doctor's clinical abilities. The team must hold these key convictions:

- The smile designer has the best interest of his or her patients at heart

- The doctor can create and deliver the outcome that is proposed

- The restorative plan includes optimal adhesive dentistry without compromise, while bringing together interdisciplinary services

Note, I did not say "without failure or mistakes"—just without excuses. No one is perfect all the time. Human error occurs. Lab miscommunication happens. Differing perceptions among and between patient, dentist, and team can all add up to clinical challenges. But when a team player holds the core belief in the dentist and team, the patient picks up on it and recognizes the value and sincerity in care planning.

Another reason the team must trust in the dentist's integrity is that patients often turn to their dental hygienists, dental assistants, and even business personnel for treatment validation and help in decision making. When patients schedule appointments, they sometimes double-check the diagnosis with the appointment coordinator just to further ensure that the work "really does need to be done." Patients commonly ask their hygienist after the dentist has left the smile studio, "Do I really need that? What would you do? Can he/she really make over my smile to look like that? How long will it last?" Wouldn't it reinforce your professionalism and the practice's aesthetic mission if, during the restorative diagnosis, the doctor restated everything the hygienist had previously discussed? The patient would no longer need to turn to the hygienist for verification. The patient would ease into case acceptance with confidence, having had the hygienist pre-diagnose and discuss restorative and aesthetic possibilities, and the dentist's diagnosis would support that pre-diagnostic assessment.

The third transformation occurs when a team player connects the patient's wants and needs with preventive and restorative actions. He or she has given the patient the knowledge and education needed to collaborate in their care plan. Knowing that you played—and will continue to play—a central role in helping patients achieve and maintain their oral health and smile goals is the ultimate burn-out buster.

Increase Awareness for Aesthetic and Restorative Services

Oral health care professionals have the chance to offer aesthetic treatment options, which, in some cases, can be life altering. Many consumer magazines have published articles and surveys that underscore the public's emphasis on looking good and feeling good. The American Academy of Cosmetic Dentistry conducted a survey in 1997 and discovered that 75 percent of the people polled believed an aesthetic smile would help their chances of career success. Additionally, there is growing literature that addresses aesthetic restorative treatment and its positive effect on patients' self-esteem and sense of well being.

Beauty and the emotional responses to it are important aspects of aesthetic and restorative dentistry. Just as you choose to wear a certain suit or outfit, adhere to a physical fitness schedule, or have straight or curly hair, we make these choices to create what we believe to be beautiful. This means that a beautiful or perfect smile means different things to different people. It may mean a disease-free smile, a sassy smile, a sexy smile, a Hollywood-white smile, or an amalgam-free smile

The key is to build interest in aesthetic and restorative services by increasing awareness. You do this by incorporating an aesthetic and restorative prediagnostic examination during every recare appointment.

Hygienists usually feel quite comfortable performing the following procedures:

- Review of medical and dental history
- Head and neck cancer screening
- Periodontal and intraoral examinations

How about performing pre-assessment on the following?

- Behavioral questions
- Nutritional input
- Occlusal/TMD evaluations
- Oral malodor
- Oral habits
- Restorative management/preservation
- Smile discrepancies

We must communicate with our patients, explaining what we're doing. Do not work in a dome of silence that is only to be disturbed when you give your lunch order! By discussing all these screenings, examinations, and fact-finding procedures, you will open up many avenues to invite the patient into the assessment. This allows patients to discuss more freely any concerns they have. By including smile analysis in our daily hygiene appointments, we are able to begin to improve our patients' appearance—not by hard-selling them, but by opening up to them the possibilities and the services your practice has to offer.

Identification of aesthetic restorations

The search for restorations that reproduce natural dentition has changed operative dentistry and dental hygiene. Adhesive materials, techniques, and proper continuing education have allowed oral health professionals to deliver and maintain various direct, semi-direct, and indirect methods. Theses definitive restorations range from a broad spectrum of composite resins to numerous ceramic materials. The aesthetic and functional results involve minimal invasive preparation, tooth reinforcement, and tooth sealing. When completed and meticulously polished, they can be virtually impossible to tell apart from adjacent dentition.

The dental hygiene process of care includes:

- Assessment
- A dental hygiene diagnosis and care plan
- Implementation
- Evaluation

The traditional assessment phase embraces health, dental and behavioral data, vital signs, oral and intraoral structures, dentition, periodontal tissue, and oral hygiene. Assessment of the dentition brings new challenges in the era of tooth-colored restorations.

Recognizing and detecting aesthetic materials and smile evaluation

Visual, clinical, intra-oral camera-phonographic, and radiographic examinations can be used to differentiate a porcelain or ceramic restoration from composite or enamel. Radiographic images can aid in the identification due to the varying radiopacities of the aesthetic materials. The most radiopaque shades are from metal (such as amalgam and gold). Composite resins containing glass filler particles (hybrids) and ceramic materials have varying radiopacities. Microfill composite resins contain only small silica particles and appear radiolucent. Conventional radiography generally shows about 16 shades of gray, but still may limit our ability to determine the restoration and tooth interface. However, newer digital imagery can show several *hundred* variations of color and may further aid a team member in the radiographic identification.

The visual and clinical examination involves a sharp explorer, mirror, dental floss, a small surgical air tip, magnification loupes, and accurately documented aesthetic treatment or computer forms. Visual identification begins by applying air to clear debris or to dry tooth surfaces. Since most composite and ceramic materials reflect, refract, absorb, or transmit light rays differently than enamel and dentin, a method known as transillumination can be used to visually distinguish restorations. This is achieved by reflecting light through the tooth from the lingual surface using a mouth mirror and a specialty or operatory light. The light source illuminates the tooth and restorative materials differently for visual recognition. In addition, by using a small surgical air-tip, the clinician can dry the tooth and gently move the gingival margin back to reveal the restorative margin. (Fig.2–2)

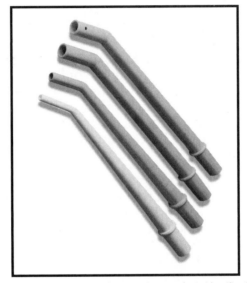

Fig. 2–2: *The 3mm opening tip may be part of an aesthetic identification armamentarium (Surg-O-Vac courtesy of Young Dental).*

Careful tactile sensitivity is essential to distinguish the restoration material and tooth structure margin. Use gentle pressure with exploratory strokes. If the margin is incorrectly identified as calcified deposit and aggressively scaled, damage to the aesthetic restoration and possible tooth structure may occur. However, if the margins were poorly finished and polished, these areas are more vulnerable to stain and bacteria accumulation. In addition, localized inflammation can result.

An aesthetic form or clinical software may be used to record the aesthetic dentistry completed and future treatment plans. Auditing the aesthetic treatment form prior to the hygiene or doctor session, and making necessary preparations, allows the clinician to work seamlessly while adding value for the patient. Remember: When the provider is prepared, the patient perceives the dental team as efficient, professional, and knowledgeable.

The explosion in the field of material technology and adhesion is revolutionizing the way dentistry is delivered. The emphasis on conservation of tooth structure, biocompatibility with gingival tissue, improved bonding with natural teeth, and cosmetic improvement has ignited this rapid development. Dental manufacturers are partnering with experts in research, academia, and private practice to develop materials with properties that will allow ease of handling, aesthetically pleasing results, durability, and low-wear resistance.

Since the restorative product *du jour* changes rapidly, the contemporary team members should continually research and learn about the newest advances in restorative and aaesthetic dentistry. This in turn will allow the hygienist, assistants, and business teams the ability to discuss treatment modalities and help guide patients to the best services for their individual clinical needs and smile goals.

Restoring a decayed tooth or replacing a defective filling can create myriad confusion concerning the best restorative products and techniques—for example, direct (placed chairside at the same appointment) or indirect (laboratory-processed, requiring a second appointment for placement); the best laboratories and philosophies of care, etc. Since there are no absolutes or best ways to treat a patient, the following are some important elements to keep in mind to aid in the ultimate success of the restorative case.

Materials selection must concur with the specific situation; the technique for tooth preparation; the restoration fabrication; the luting/bonding agent; the restorative dentist's skill, judgment, and expertise, and—in situations involving indirect restorative systems—the laboratory technicians' skill, judgment, and expertise.

Direct materials

Composite-based resin materials contain an organic resin base and inorganic glass filler particles. Composite resins are usually classified according to the filler particle size. Macrofill composites have a particle size ranging between 10 and 100 microns;

microfill particles can range from 1 to .1 microns. Hybrid composites exhibit a combination of sizes ranging from 1 to .04 microns. The inorganic filler particle size (and degree of filler loading) determines the physical properties and clinical characteristics of the material. A few examples of composite physical and mechanical properties include polymerization shrinkage/stress, hardness, bond strength, fluorescence, consistency and handling, shades, and depth of cure.

Polymerization shrinkage (the metamorphosis of the material from a gel to a solid state via light or mechanical initiation) continues to be an issue in adhesion dentistry. The complexities surrounding polymerization—how a material will shrink, how shrinkage will affect the adhesive bond of the material to the tooth structure, the light source and rate of curing most clinically appropriate—play out in the research and in scientific journals. The main concern with excessive material shrinkage is that it may contribute to marginal breakdowns.

Disease Free Soft Tissue, Before Smile Enhancement

To achieve and manage healthy tissue, a set protocol needs to be established for care prior to the provisional stage of a smile redesign. In addition, hygiene protocols are a necessity during the provisional phase and after definitive restorations are placed.

Composite resin systems can be used in the restoration of anterior or posterior teeth. Anterior composites (usually microfills) can mimic enamel, are highly aesthetic, have a high polishability, resist wear, and leave the control and artistry to the dentist. Microfills can be used to replace enamel in class III, IV, and V restorations, diastema closures, and hand-sculptured veneers.

Posterior composites (typically hybrids) are indicated for the restoration of small-to-medium defects in back teeth, and can also be used for the replacement of broken or lost fillings. Though hybrid material can be used for anterior restorations, hybrid composite materials possess strength and polishability and are commonly used for posterior areas.

These restorations are technique- sensitive and usually require the dentist to take a hands-on continuing education program to learn the correct bonding steps. If performed correctly, and in a clean and dry operating field, they can require less tooth structure removal when compared with amalgam, and can strengthen the tooth. The recognized placement techniques for composite resins are horizontal, oblique, vertical, bulk, and incremental.

Commonly, the restoring dentist will use an incremental layering and polymerization technique. Composite resins up to 2 mm (the depth of each layer in the incremental technique) can be appropriately cured with standard curing lights to help prevent polymerization shrinkage. Most documented research concludes that efficient light curing requires a curing device with a minimum energy output of 400mW/cm2. Other types of composite resin systems include micro-hybrids, resin/glass ionomers, flowable composites, packable composites, and compomors.

Clinical examination will show that microfill composites, when finished and polished precisely, are very glossy and feel smooth to the tip of an applied explorer. An additional microfill category, reinforced microfills, may be used in additional enamel replacement areas. So, if you are unsure of the material (hybrid composites or microfill composites), remember that hybrids have a combination of large filler particles (glass) for strength and smaller particles (silica) for polishability and aesthetics. Hybrids may cause more of a drag when an explorer is drawn across the surface. They can easily be mistaken for microfills, but cannot be polished as effortlessly.

Small particle composites are considered obsolete as a restorative material because they have a rough surface. However, many patients may still have serviceable small particle restorations. Clinically, they are unmistakable because of the rough feeling when navigating the surface with an explorer. Due to their early introduction, a majority of small particle composites contain quartz as a filler particle. Black lines may appear after an explorer crosses a small particle composite resin when the instrument scratches the quartz.

Indirect materials

Indirect restorative systems continually increase in options and popularity. Indirect restoratives are fabricated in a laboratory and cemented or bonded to natural tooth structure. This procedure requires excellent communication and collaboration between the restoring dentist and the laboratory technician who is fabricating the restoration. To further enhance a dental team's understanding of indirect restoration fabrication, a field trip to a referring laboratory may be advised. While visiting and touring the laboratory, one can gain insights to the skill and expertise needed to make these restorations. This experience can translate into greater confidence in the team's ability to create value for such treatments, which in turn can increase restorative and aesthetic enrollment and case acceptance when discussing possibilities with patients.

Ceramic materials are the foundation for indirect restoration placement. They can be used for inlays, onlays, veneers, metal-free crowns, and crowns with metal substructures. Since many hygienists are most familiar with porcelain (specifically feldspathic), one may wonder why the ceramic category has emerged so quickly. Porcelain—especially roughened or nonpolished porcelain—historically performs very aggressively against opposing teeth. Lucite-based ceramic products not only can mirror natural tooth structure in appearance, fluorescence, and translucency, but do not abrade the opposing dentition as quickly as feldspathic.

Advances of Metal-Free Bonded Indirect Restorations vs. Metal

- *No metal to reflect light*
- *Creates invisible margin*
- *Decreases opaqueness*
- *More natural translucency*
- *Supragingival margin*

Ceramic categories can be broken down into ceramics bonded, ceramometal restorations, and a variety of types that may not fit into a particular category.

When an explorer glides over the glass-hard surface of porcelain or ceramic materials, a "scratchy" sensation can be felt—and probably heard. Surfaces retain a glossy finish if they retained their initial shine during seating and finishing, if the restoration was refinished when adjustments were warranted, *i.e.* if abusive patient care approaches were eliminated, and if proper clinician management was maintained during professional sessions.

The first step in understanding and identifying aesthetic dentistry is developing a clear understanding and first hand knowledge. It's hard to spotlight the smile if too many demands keep hygienists from exploring unfamiliar solutions. Consider the opening lines in a A.A. Milne's classic, *Winnie the Pooh*, and try to avoid a similar professional fate:

"Here is Edward Bear, coming downstairs now, bump, bump, bump, on the back of his head, behind Christopher Robin. It is, as far as he knows, the only way of coming downstairs, but sometimes he feels that there really is another way, if only he could stop bumping for a moment and think of it."

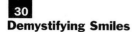
Team Smile Screening

Since a smile evaluation involves subjective, objective, and clinical investigations, it can be kick started with the patient completing a written questionnaire. This may provide a hygienist or clinical assistant a beginning point to engage in an interactive, co-assessment discussion that reflects on appearance-enhancing dentistry and its impact on health.

A team member can then look at other variables of the smile stage. This involves all supporting structures (facial abbreviations, lips, gingival tissue, osseous tissue, and teeth). Begin with the lip line—at rest and during a wide smile. Does the patient show little or an obvious space between the maxillary posterior teeth and inner cheek, buccal corridor? Does the profile exhibit a wide smile, displaying the pre-molar and molar regions (Julia Roberts-style) that should be included in the smile redesign?

The gingival tissue forum includes color, absence of disease, amount of gingiva showing ("gummy smile"), and the amount of attached gingiva. Hard tissue can be evaluated for symmetry, thickness, and amount of bone loss. The teeth can be evaluated for mobility, tooth color, size, shape, position, inclination, and arch position.

In addition, the exploration can uncover the integrity of previous dentistry (or lack thereof), dark lines in the gingival margins (sign of biological width violation), breakdown of previous tooth-colored restorations, opaque crowns, and/or missing teeth. The principles of occlusion—including grinding, clenching, incisal guidance, and temporomandibular joint problems—also need a careful evaluation. Detailed assessments may also include diagnostic study casts, updated radiographs, full-mouth periodontal assessment, and intra-oral and extra-oral photography.

In order to always remain attentive to the patient's concept of a beautiful smile and keep his or her participation in the process, an intra oral camera, computer imaging, and an educational system are paramount during case presentations. An intra-oral camera can be used for education and patient enlightenment during the data-collection stage. Computer imaging can portray the desired appearance for the patient prior to the beginning of any treatment, while an educational system can further clarify any remaining clinical questions. An office protocol using these technologies during the team smile evaluation and comprehensive-aesthetic examinations should be revisited or developed.

By now, some clinicians may be thinking, "Why do hygienists or assistants need to know all this information about restorations and smile designs?" Answer: What we see is what we look for. What we look for is what we know. Professionals never limit their educational opportunities!

Team players must also establish measurable goals in their desire to perform smile evaluations. Saying—out loud, at a team meeting—that you will start to use the intra-oral camera and the smile-evaluation form, or to talk about adhesive procedures is an admirable, yet indefinable goal. Committing to using the intra-oral camera with at least three patients in the morning, giving a smile evaluation form to all three-month recare patients—all of these actions create *focus.* These actions can be measured, changed, and championed.

There should be harmony between the dentist and the clinical teams concerning responsibilities placed on them when it comes to pre-framing smile evaluations. Once the guidelines have been discussed and agreed upon by all professionals, a specific model and process can be implemented in the assessment phase of the dental hygiene process of care. This will ensure the level at which all team members feel confident in performing such data collection and evaluations.

Sound Bites of Aesthetic Concepts

Defining what aesthetics means involves—

- Working with the patient to define mutual goals
- Remembering that in dentistry and dental hygiene, *the patient* is the most important individual when developing aesthetic treatments

Why patients seek oral care

Economic. From television actors to plumbers, confidence in one's appearance can be essential to success. It has been shown many times that bias favors the more attractive individual.

Social. A good self-image is enhanced by an attractive smile. Society has become increasingly aware of the desirability of a pleasing smile. What is considered attractive may vary in different social groups. Again, the media image has a strong influence.

Psychological. Patients with unrealistic or ill-defined goals may never be pleased. Many of us are familiar with patients who, after whitening their teeth, have become whitening junkies, regardless of the appearance or shade of their teeth. Patients seeking change without well-defined goals may never be satisfied.

Traumatic injury. From a small chip of an incisal edge to the major defects caused by an automobile accident, oral trauma may require oral care.

Developmental anomalies. Atypical dental development can be reason enough for aesthetic dental care—such as anodontia, oligodontia, twinning, peg lateral incisors, etc.

Disease. Whether systemic (tetracycline discoloration, flouro-sis) or local (caries), a disease process may necessitate aesthetic restoration.

What does the patient want?

This must be determined as early in patient care as possible. It is essential to establish two-way communication channels. Ask the patient, "How can I help you?"—and then listen!

Establish what the patient wants from oral care. When you think you know what the patient has said, rephrase it to ensure that you are communicating—not just mirroring. Learn the patient's values and concepts. Patients may be very specific or very vague in their requests for dental and hygiene care.

Patients must also be brought to the understanding of the difference between aesthetic and purely cosmetic restorations. When there is no need-based indication for a restoration, and the patient insists on smile design, he or she must be made aware of the biologic price that is paid when the tooth-tissue interface is violated, or when tooth structure is unnecessarily removed.

Remember, people now live longer, and this places more stringent requirements upon the longevity of the restoration. Elective procedures require that the patient be completely informed about the possible negative consequences—as well as the benefits—of the treatments, and this recognition should be documented in writing before therapy begins.

What does the patient need?

A thorough examination—including complete dental and medical histories, extra-oral and intra-oral examinations, diagnostic casts, photographs, diagnosis, and connected dental hygiene and restorative treatment plans—is essential before any care is contemplated. It is crucial to gather complete and correct data before making any diagnosis or planning any care.

What is the dental team's ability?

The patient may require services or opinions for a number of considerations that may include orthodontic services, periodontics, oral and maxillofacial surgical options, and/or prosthodontics. Consultation with dental laboratory technicians, plastic and reconstructive surgery, and psychological or nutritional counseling may be required. Medical professionals may become involved. Other specialties may be consulted or enlisted to meet patient needs and desires.

Behavioral questions to consider and document

Does the patient:

- Use tobacco? Type? Have interest in a cessation program?

- Chew or bite lips?

- Chew or bite cheeks?

- Suck fingers or thumb?

- Chew ice?

- Hold pins or needles in mouth?

- Chew pencils, pens, or any hard objects?

- Chew or hold eye/sun glasses in mouth?

> **Team Smile Design Protocols**
>
> *Shared and understood by the team and implemented on a consistent basis can lead to increased aesthetic and restorative discussions and acceptance.*

- Play a musical instrument that requires holding the instrument with teeth?

- Use toothpicks or similar wood or plastic cleaning devices?

- Keep tongue thrust against teeth?

- Place tongue in the space between teeth?

- Grind or clench teeth?

- Use a bite/night guard?

Mouth malodor: Consider and document

- Is the patient aware of his or her breath odor?

- Does the patient notice a bad taste in his or her mouth?

- Has the patient ever had treatments for bad breath?

- Is the patient's tongue frequently coated with white or yellowish deposits?

- Has someone pointed out the patient's bad breath to him or her?

- Has the patient's breath ever interfered with the ability to communicate at work?

- Is the patient on a special diet?

- Does the patient suffer from postnasal drip, hay fever, or other allergy-related symptoms?

Clinically . . . consider:

- Is mouth odor present?

- Degree of malodor:

  - Questionable odor

  - Slight odor

  - Moderate odor

  - Strong odor

  - Severe odor

Xerostomia: Consider and document

According to Laclede, Inc. (www.laclede.com), more than 80 percent of adults suffer from dry mouth. This condition is caused by a number of factors, including stress, depression, and medication side effects. (More than 400 prescription and over-the-counter medications cause xerostomia, including antidepressants and antihistamines). Symptoms may also arise as a result of aging, radiation therapy, chemotherapy, diabetes, kidney dialysis, Sjogrens Syndrome, lupus, smoking, alcohol, HIV/AIDS, cystic fibrosis, Prader Willi Syndrome, and vitamin deficiencies.

Dry mouth results from the body's inability to create sufficient amounts of salvia. Without saliva, the mouth has no healthy balance of bacteria to fight the harmful germs that try to enter the body.

Dry mouth is a serious problem, with potential for causing long-term damage to teeth, including oral infections, gingivitis, and compromising the long-term predictability of smile design outcomes and definitive restorative therapies.

Does the patient:

- Suffer from constant thirst?
- Suffer any dryness or cracking of the mouth, lips, throat, or nose?
- Have difficulty in speaking, chewing, or swallowing foods?
- Have a persistent dry cough?
- Change in texture of the tongue?
- Find it difficult to tolerate spicy or acidic foods?

Clinically . . . consider:

- Dry chapped lips
- Tender or swollen parotid glands
- Tender or swollen submandibular glands
- Tender or swollen around ears
- Desiccated mucosa surfaces

- Red, fissured, denuded, or shiny tongue
- Thick saliva, lack of saliva, saliva of an opaque or yellowish color, or absence of a saliva pool on the bottom of the mouth
- Caries involving cervical surfaces and or incisal edges

Diet analysis: Consider and document

Does the patient consume:

- Coffee or tea, with or without sugar?
- Dark-pigmented drinks, sugar or sugar-free?
- Drinks high in citric or phosphoric acid?
- Sugar or sugar-free candy, gums, or mints? (Xyletol, Sorbital)

Team Smile Assessment Checklist (Fig. 2-3 page 41)

First impression

- Intra-oral examination
- Extra-oral examination
- Oral cancer examination

Facial Analysis

- Facial asymmetry may inhibit the adherence to some smile-design criteria. (Fig. 2–3: Part 2)
- Normal occlusion: orthognathic profile
- Class I malocclusion: orthognathic profile
- Class II: retrognathic profile
- Class III: prognathic profile

Jaw Relationship

Maxilla. Normal, retruded, protruded

Mandible. Normal, retruded, protruded

Vertical. Normal, overclosed

Lip in repose. Lip appearance during relaxation (Note: Tooth position can affect lip position, and arch relationships can have a great bearing on the dental appearance during relaxation. The extreme example is the inability of the lips to cover the teeth—lip incompetency—usually seen in Class II malocclusions or in bimaxillary protrusion. (Fig. 2–3, Part 2)

Ideal smile line. Maxillary anterior incisal edges should be framed by mandibular lip when smiling. The smile exposes almost all of the maxillary central incisors just to the gingival line, revealing the tips of the papillae. (Fig. 2–3, Part 3)

Low lip line. Revealing no or minimum gingival tissue when smiling. (Fig. 2–3, Part 3A-C)

High lip line. All teeth and gum tissue are exposed when smiling (>2mm., i.e. gummy smile) (Fig. 2–3, Part 3A-C)

Reverse smile line. Canines appear longer than central incisors (Fig. 2–3, Part 3A-C)

Display of teeth. How many maxillary teeth are exposed during a full smile (maxillary, mandibular, viewed directly from the front and sides?) (Fig. 2–3, Part 3D)

Shape. Square, tapered, ovoid

Shade of aesthetic zone. Involves value, hue, chroma, and polychromatic variables. Since no tooth is monochromatic—many apparent traits are darker chroma near the gingival third, while the incisal edge shows a transparency—evaluate centrals, incisals, canines, pre-molars, and molars.

Attributes of the aesthetic zone

Incisal edge display. The amount of tooth exhibited (tooth show)

Incisal edge. Mamelon development, prominent edge detail, moderate edge detail, smooth edge detail, chipped

Facial surface. High texture, medium texture, smooth texture (Fig. 2–3, Part 5)

Midline-vertical. Invisible line from the forehead to the chin. The two central incisors should be at right angles to the horizontal plane and parallel to the midline of the face. (Fig. 2–3, Part 3E-F). Note:

- midline is vertical with centrals (drops straight down from the papilla located between the two maxillary centrals)

- midline is right of centrals

- midline is left of centrals

Axial alignment/inclination. Compares the vertical alignment of maxillary teeth to the central vertical midline. If one draws a line from the gingival apex to the center of the incisal edge or incisal apex of the cuspids, the centrals are the straightest to the midline with a gradually increasing mesial inclination back to the first bicuspids. (Fig. 2–3, Part 4C)

Incisal embrasures. The contact points (and subsequent spaces between the teeth at the incisal edge) from the centrals to the canines should increase in size or depth and move apically as they proceed posteriorly.

Principle of golden proportion. Identifies what the eye can already see from the frontal view. It incorporates a mathematical ratio between the widths of the centrals, laterals, and canines. (Fig. 2–3, Part 4A-B)

Size proportion of central (dominance). Generally, a 3:5 (.8 to 1.0), or a range of 75-percent to 80-percent width-to-length ratio is accepted. This means that if a tooth is 10mm long, it should be 7.5mm to 8mm wide.

Some smile designers align themselves with the perception that shorter teeth make the smile appear older, while longer teeth may give the smile a more youthful appearance.

Buccal corridor. The buccal corridor (or negative space) refers to what is visible between the corners of the mouth and the facial surfaces of the maxillary teeth. (Fig. 2–3, Part 3G)

Narrow buccal corridor. Perception is a "mouthful" of teeth

Wide buccal corridor. Perception is "darkness," or too little teeth shown.

Soft-tissue aesthetics

Periodontal health. Generally includes healthy supportive tissues, perfect tissue architecture, stippled gingiva, manageable sulcus, and appropriate bone level. Some common conditions that could affect the manageability of health and are no longer acceptable due to compromising the long-term predictability, which would jeopardize the success of the new smile. Be sure to:

- Look beyond the no-bleeding guideline

- Provide early treatment intervention

- Evaluate the amount of attached gingival

Gingival gradation. Teeth get shorter from the cuspids back. If there is a discrepancy in the gradation or disharmony in the linear perspective from the canines' posteriorly anterioposterior progression, it may detract from the new smile.

Gingival symmetry. Bilateral mirror image to each other (Fig. 2–3, Part 4D)

Gingival height. The gingival height is the position or level at the cervical. Generally, the laterals incisors are 1mm to 2mm gingivally shorter than centrals and cuspids.

Gingival form. The gingival tissue form contributes to or detracts from aesthetics. Relative tissue height, recession, or poor contour all play a role in the aesthetic picture. Inadequate gingival contours may be reconstructed with surgical or laser recontouring and or grafts. Aesthetics begins with the soft tissues!

Cervical embrasures: This darkens interproximally (dark triangles).

Intra-arch and inter-arch relationships

Evaluate for:

- Non-carious lesions

- Caries

- Chips

- Crossbite

- Diastema (The attractiveness or unattractiveness of a diastema is a matter of personal opinion.)

- Edge to edge
- Facets and wear patterns
- Fracture
- Missing teeth
- Mobility
- Overerupted
- Recession
- Rotation
- Tipping
  - Labioversion
  - Linguversion
- Undererupted
- Maximum opening

Temporal mandibular joints

Consider, and ask your patients if they have had or have:

- Sounds occurring during open or close
- Clicking
- Crepitis
- History of locking
- Muscle tenderness
- Popping
- Protrusive movement
- Sagittal movement
- Swelling

Esthetic Evaluation

Patient _____ Examiner _____ Date ____ / ____ / ____

1. Effective Questions (E.Q.)

A. If there was anything you could change about your smile, what would it be?

_____
_____
_____
_____
_____

B. Do you like the Media Image of "Perfectly Straight, White" looking teeth, or are you content with "Healthy, Clean, Natural" looking teeth?

❏ Media Image   ❏ Natural Looking

C. History of esthetic change.

_____
_____
_____
_____
_____

D. Previous Records...
Do you have any previous photographs of your smile to aid in your Esthetic Treatment Planning?

❏ Yes   ❏ No

2. Facial Analysis

A. Full Smile
1. Interpupillary Line to Occlusal Plane
   ❏ Parallel   ❏ Canted Right   ❏ Canted Left

2. Midline Relationship of Teeth (Central Incisor) to Face (Philtrum)
   ❏ Symmetric   ❏ Right of Center   ❏ Left of Center

3. Relationship of Lips to Face (Lip Symmetry)
   ❏ Symmetric   ❏ Right   ❏ Left

Fig. 2–3a: *Aesthetic evaluation form, created by Jonathan B. Levine, D.M.D., and David Gane, D.M.D. All rights reserved.*

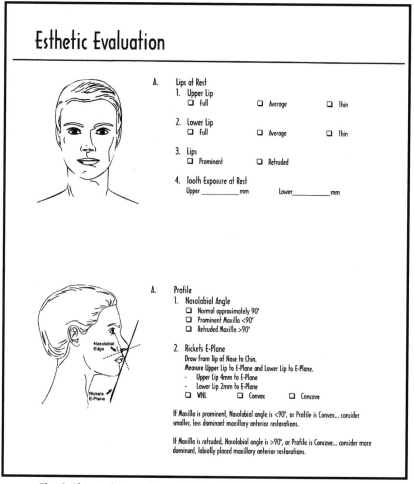

Esthetic Evaluation

A. Lips at Rest
1. Upper Lip
   ☐ Full ☐ Average ☐ Thin

2. Lower Lip
   ☐ Full ☐ Average ☐ Thin

3. Lips
   ☐ Prominent ☐ Retruded

4. Tooth Exposure at Rest
   Upper _____ mm Lower _____ mm

A. Profile
1. Nasolabial Angle
   ☐ Normal approximately 90°
   ☐ Prominent Maxilla <90°
   ☐ Retruded Maxilla >90°

2. Rickets E-Plane
   Draw from Tip of Nose to Chin.
   Measure Upper Lip to E-Plane and Lower Lip to E-Plane.
   - Upper Lip 4mm to E-Plane
   - Lower Lip 2mm to E-Plane
   ☐ WNL ☐ Convex ☐ Concave

If Maxilla is prominent, Nasolabial angle is <90°, or Profile is Convex... consider smaller, less dominant maxillary anterior restorations.

If Maxilla is retruded, Nasolabial angle is >90°, or Profile is Concave... consider more dominant, labially placed maxillary anterior restorations.

Fig. 2–3b: *Aesthetic evaluation form, created by Jonathan B. Levine, D.M.D., and David Gane, D.M.D. All rights reserved.*

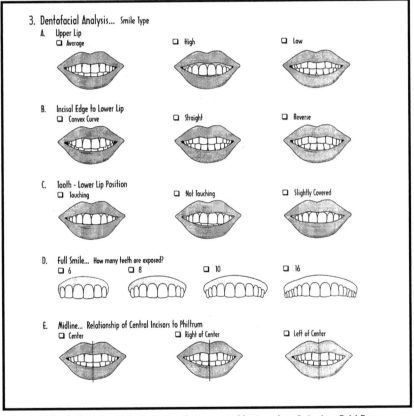

Fig. 2–3c: *Aesthetic evaluation form, created by Jonathan B. Levine, D.M.D., and David Gane, D.M.D. All rights reserved.*

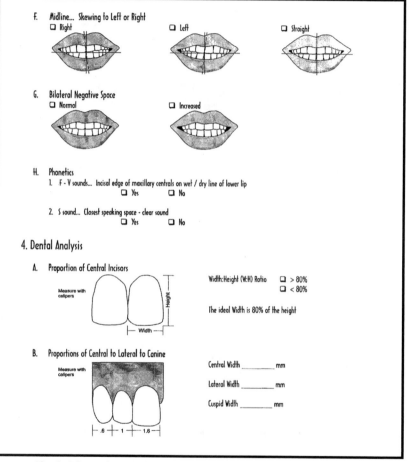

Fig. 2–3d: *Aesthetic evaluation form, created by Jonathan B. Levine, D.M.D., and David Gane, D.M.D. All rights reserved.*

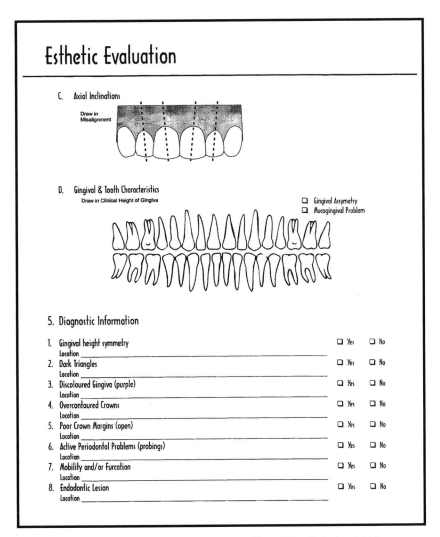

Esthetic Evaluation

C. Axial Inclinations

Draw in
Misalignment

D. Gingival & Tooth Characteristics
Draw in Clinical Height of Gingiva

☐ Gingival Assymetry
☐ Mucogingival Problem

5. Diagnostic Information

		Yes	No
1.	Gingival height symmetry	☐ Yes	☐ No
	Location		
2.	Dark Triangles	☐ Yes	☐ No
	Location		
3.	Discoloured Gingiva (purple)	☐ Yes	☐ No
	Location		
4.	Overcontoured Crowns	☐ Yes	☐ No
	Location		
5.	Poor Crown Margins (open)	☐ Yes	☐ No
	Location		
6.	Active Periodontal Problems (probings)	☐ Yes	☐ No
	Location		
7.	Mobility and/or Furcation	☐ Yes	☐ No
	Location		
8.	Endodontic Lesion	☐ Yes	☐ No
	Location		

Fig. 2–3e: *Aesthetic evaluation form, created by Jonathan B. Levine, D.M.D., and David Gane, D.M.D. All rights reserved.*

Esthetic Evaluation

9. Occlusion - wear facets/incisal wear ☐ Yes ☐ No
   Location _____
10. Continuous progression from canine distally (coincidence of curves) ☐ Yes ☐ No
    Location _____
11. Flared Teeth ☐ Yes ☐ No
    Location _____
12. Diastema ☐ Yes ☐ No
    Location _____
13. Overlapped Teeth ☐ Yes ☐ No
    Location _____
14. Chipped Teeth ☐ Yes ☐ No
    Location _____
15. Discoloured Teeth ☐ Yes ☐ No
    Location _____
16. Surface Texture... Smooth ☐ Yes ☐ No
    ☐ Light ☐ Medium ☐ High

6. Diagnostic Information Checklist

   ☐ Esthetic Evaluation Form
   ☐ Study Casts... Diagnostic Wax-ups
   ☐ Computer Imaging or Similar Visualization Tool

Fig. 2–3f: *Aesthetic evaluation form, created by Jonathan B. Levine, D.M.D., and David Gane, D.M.D. All rights reserved.*

Maximizing Lab Communication to Generate the Awe-Inspiring Smile!

by Trish Jones, R.D.H., B.S.
Aurum Ceramic Dental Laboratories

Imagine a patient sitting in the dental chair, full of anticipation for that new smile the team is ready to try in. The dentist hands the patient a mirror and waits for the patient to endorse the beauty. Everyone's heart is pounding. The restorations look great and we await the patient's response. The patient holds up the mirror and evaluates the porcelain teeth. "I thought they would be whiter. And why do the front teeth look like they are more to the right?" inquires the patient.

A sigh of disappointment, as your heart falls into your stomach. You, as the clinical assistant, hygienist, or administrative personnel, know the patient is not happy. Our minds race to try to determine what went wrong. Did the lab technician not read the prescription? How could the midline be off center? Yes, we all know what I am talking about. We have all witnessed those cases where the shade is way off, the crowns do not fit, etc., and wondered if it was the laboratory's janitor who actually worked on the case!

Before you ponder any further, sit back and think about how you communicated the critical facts about the case to the laboratory.

Was the laboratory informed of that midline shift? Could the current shade-taking process have been improved? Did we "show" the laboratory the shades and characterization we really wanted? Usually, when a case does not go as planned, it is not the result of poor laboratory skills, but rather a lack of communication skills between the laboratory and dental office. *Missing vital information is often the culprit!*

Do you consider your laboratory technician/ceramist part of your dental crew? If not, you should! Your dental laboratory technician/ceramist shares an integral part in producing outstanding aesthetic results. It takes meticulous communication and teamwork between the dental team and the laboratory to create living dental art. (Figs.2–4, 2–5)

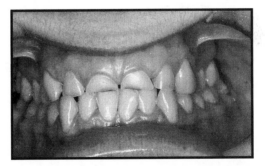

Fig. 2–4: *Pretreatment photo, courtesy of Scott Brody, D.D.S.*

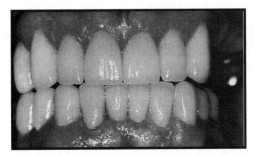

Fig. 2–5: *Maxillary definitive treatment photo, dentistry courtesy of Scott Brody, D.D.S.; lab work by Aurum Ceramic.*

There is no such thing as too much information!

An aesthetic smile design case necessitates pertinent documentation. This documentation includes:

- Adequate impression of the preparation with a 360-degree view of margins

- Correct bite registration, including stick bite to verify that the incisal edge of centrals is parallel with the interpupilary line of the eyes

- Indication of stump shades of the prepped teeth

- Utilization of the appropriate shade guide for blending shades together for a more natural appearance

- Type of restorations requested such as crowns, veneers, inlays, etc.

- Type of aesthetic material (such as Empress porcelain, Critical+, etc.)

- Indications of any bridges and pontic design

- Detailed instructions on the characteristics necessary to fabricate all porcelain restorations, such as level of translucency, surface anatomy, incisal check lines, and halo

- Desired smile design such as enhanced, softened, natural, etc.

- Desired length of centrals (so the ceramist may create the golden proportion of the smile)

- Photos of pre-operative teeth, preps, and provisionals

- Pre-operative models

- Preference of articulator

- Detailed color map and lab prescription of the above mentioned items (Figs. 2–6, 2–7)

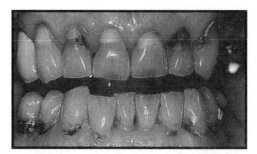

Fig. 2–6: *Pretreatment photo, courtesy of Wayne Myles, D.D.S.*

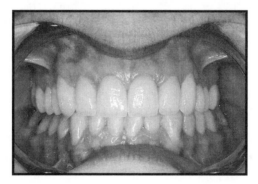

Fig.2–7: *Post-treatment photo, dentistry courtesy of Wayne Myles, D.D.S.;
lab work by Aurum Ceramic.*

Most likely you are thinking, "Why do I need to know about this?" Team members—the clinical assistant, hygienist, and administrative personnel—play a crucial role in the success of any aesthetic case, as liaison among the dentist, the patient, and the laboratory. Never underestimate your expertise, abilities, or importance! Often, the team member follows up on the case with the laboratory. It is an essential fundamental responsibility for the dental team to understand what it takes to get restorations back from the lab as indicated.

When team members grow their knowledge of laboratory repertoire, they increase their value to the dental practice through their ability to discuss aesthetics with the patient. All things considered, in the end, what makes the patient happy is what matters. Hence, formulate awe-inspiring smiles by providing details, details, and more details! Those details include degrees of characteristics and shading.

Characteristics include surface anatomy, incisal characteristics, translucency, halo, and checklines. These characteristics give life and brilliance to otherwise artificial teeth. Inform the ceramist of the level desired for anatomy, incisal detail, and translucency—light, medium, or heavy. Indicate if a halo and/or checklines are desired. (A halo replicates light reflection on the incisal edge, and checklines can be added to mature the look of the restorations.)

One factor that team members can influence is shade preference. Remember, you aspire to grant the patient his or her wishes. Admittedly, our worst fear is that the patient walks out the door with a Chicklet smile, or a Game Show Host appearance! Put aside your trepidations and do what you can to accommodate the patient while achieving your goal of creating the radiant smile the patient so desires. A resourceful tool you can use to convey details is a color map.

A color map is a detailed illustration of the shading and characteristics of the teeth to be restored. You can actually use different-colored markers to draw out where you want the shades on the restorations. It may sound like first-grade coloring class, but realize that ceramists process visual information rapidly. Since natural teeth are not monochromatic, and are usually a shade darker at the gingival third, it is recommended to blend at least two shades for a natural appearance and up to four shades, if desired.

It all depends on the level of aesthetics you desire. Certain laboratories have special teams of ceramists who work on advanced cosmetic smile design cases—and most of these laboratories utilize the color map technique. If you are unsure whether your lab makes use of this system—ask!

Several shade guides are available, depending on the aesthetic material used. Maximum results can be ascertained by using the corresponding shade guide with the aesthetic material. For example, the Chromascope shade guide corresponds with Empress porcelain. They also provide a bleach-shade guide for those patients who have previously whitened their teeth. The Vita-Lumin shade guide ("vita shade guide") that has been used for many years is universal. Special shades guides, such as the stump shade guide, are used for taking shades of the prepped teeth, thus establishing the "stump shade."

For the patient, shade selection is critical; as a team member, you can greatly assist the process.

Universal shade-taking guidelines

1. What does the patient want—natural-appearing or bright white? Finding this out will help determine the base shade of the restorations. Next, blend the subsequent shade darker than the base shade at the cervical. You may even want to blend two-to-three shades in addition to the base shade.

2. What is the patient's complexion and hair color? Restorations may appear lighter on those with dark hair and dark/olive complexions as compared with the same shade on those with blonde hair and fair complexions.

3. Make sure the stump shade-prepped teeth are hydrated (prior to final impression). This will help the laboratory determine the opacity of the base porcelain (ingot). If the prepped teeth are dark, a more opaque porcelain ingot will cover up the darkness.

4. Drape the patient with a neutral gray bib or towel when taking the shade. It neutralizes the eyes' color perception.

5. Utilize color-corrected lighting. Shades will appear different under daylight, incandescent light, and fluorescent light.

6. Send photos of the patient (pre-operative), the stump shade next to prepped teeth, and the provisionals. This process is the best way to convey any midline shift or canting, or correction of gingival contours. It also helps the ceramist put a face to the artwork they are creating!

When it comes to creating vital, life-like restorations, the ceramist is an artist. But the dentist and team members bequeath the canvas, the colors, and the details of the portrait to be reinvented by the ceramist. Envision the dental team providing everything except the patient!

For optimal results, allow sufficient time for this dental artwork to be crafted. Eight to ten units usually require at least 10 working days, on average—possibly more. Special techniques are applied to smile design restorations that require a few more steps and a little more time. The final result is worth the wait! When the patient is profoundly delighted by the brilliant smile, it is conclusive proof that the dental team and the lab team have successfully corresponded on the same goal: maximum communication, generating breathtaking results! (Figs. 2–8, 2–9)

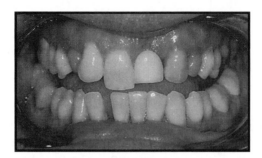

Fig. 2–8: *Pretreatment photo, courtesy of Tara Hardin, D.D.S.*

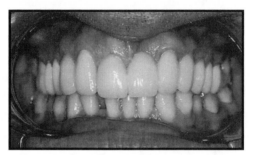

Fig. 2–9: Anterior post-treatment photo, dentistry courtesy of Tara Hardin, D.D.S.; lab work by Aurum Ceramic.

Kids Should Be Seen with Happy Smiles

Dental teams can play a role in uncovering any compelling smile issues that may be affecting their pediatric patients. A lot of children will not volunteer their concerns, especially if they are tied to their self esteem. Nor will they open up if they have expressed feelings in the past that have not been validated. Do not begin such a thread in a manner that will create even more self doubt! Creating an environment that is safe and nonjudgmental will allow the youth to express any concerns he or she may be having with their teeth.

The atmosphere should also be without sarcasm. Do not say, " Do you have a date for the prom yet? If Dr. Jones gets rid of those brown spots on your front teeth, you might have a chance!" Instead, as aesthetic practitioners, we need to employ some of the same communication principles we use with our adult patients. For instance, one might say "Johnny, as part of the dental hygiene sessions in this office, I will be performing a smile assessment. You know that we are in the smile business, so it is my privilege to make sure that everyone who visits me is happy about his or her smile. How do you feel about your smile?" In this way, the child will likely be more relaxed, knowing that he or she is not being singled out, and aware that all patients will undergo these questions and assessments.

It may take a few hygiene sessions and some rapport building until the child feels comfortable sharing insights or answering your gentle, open-ended cosmetic queries. When and if it does occur, encourage this behavior and validate the concerns. "Johnny, I appreciate you being able to share with me that you are unhappy with the brown spot on your front tooth. If something could be done to get rid of the brown spot, would you be interested in hearing about it? Let's discuss your concerns with Dr. Jones when she comes in for your examination today. And then we can talk to your parents and create a situation in which everyone wins."

The smile design areas that may be incorporated and evaluated during the pediatric visit include:

- Discoloration of teeth: brown, white, yellow, and orange stain caused by developmental disturbances

- Trauma- or medication-induced enamel hypoplasia, fluorosis, and genetic pigment distributions

- Congenitally missing anterior teeth

- Diastema

- Fused teeth

- Malformed teeth, such as a peg lateral

Treatment options for discoloration may be based on the ideology of the discoloration, the depth of the stain into the enamel, and the patient's age. A cocktail of techniques may include nightguard whitening, microabrasion, and resin composite veneers. The research is not well documented on the effects that carbamide peroxide has on the development of permanent teeth. Some studies caution that younger teeth may be more susceptible to sensitivity from the whitening agent due to the larger pulp chambers generally found in young dentitions. A modified version could be developed, wherein the patient is more closely monitored and the team utilizes a low-percentage agent, high-concentrated neutral sodium fluoride tray applications, and/or a daily protocol is replaced with every-other and/or every third-day treatments.

Microabrasion can also be used to eliminate enamel stains. Enamel microabrasion has become accepted as a conservative method of improving the appearance of teeth with superficial demineralization and decalcification defects. The procedure can be done without anesthesia and can be accomplished by chemical, mechanical, or a combination of the two methods. It can, however, leave the tooth rough, and it may be necessary, in some cases, to place a composite resin and/or a veneer over the enamel surface to restore any lost contour, create the desired color, and/or a polished surface. Additional measures that involve resin composites may utilize conservative bonded veneers. A conservative no prep approach (which assures reversibility) can be used to correct minimal malformations or gross discolorations. Another appearance-related option is modified orthodontic appliances that can be used as fixed bridgework for avulsed primary teeth as a glued-in alternative to removable, denture-type appliances.

Instead of reaching for amalgam as a posterior restoration for repairing decayed or fractured teeth, try a modified resin composite (compomer). Research shows that compomers can be placed without etching. This material may provide an advantage when "as quick as possible" is the goal (especially with children). Even though it lacks the wear resistance of other composites (and that should be a consideration on case selection), it may be a non-issue in primary teeth. Lastly, componers are fluoride releasing, and that can further benefit a child whose self-care may be less than meticulous.

Early identification of possible inclinations that may promote future aesthetic concerns should also be integrated into the hygiene assessment and self-care dialogue with the child, as well as parents/guardians. Your aesthetic eyes could recognize and document:

- Clenching or grinding habits

- Excessive fluoride consumption

- Caution when prescribing an antibiotic from the tetracycline family

- Making sure children wear protective mouth guards
- Avoidance of cavity-producing beverages and food (soda, sugar treats)
- Delayed eruption patterns or crowding

Children's Self-Care or Self-Prophy

Dr. Bob Barkley practiced dentistry and influenced many clinicians with his physiological clarity in regard to treating patients, until he was killed in a private plane crash in 1976.

He championed the concept that children are physiologically incapable of effectively cleaning their teeth (due to underdeveloped motor skills) until they are between 9 and 11 years old. Until that time, he believed, parents hold a major responsibility for removing plaque on a daily basis and creating the expectation that cleaning one's teeth on a daily basis is as normal a part of normal behavior as sleeping or breathing.

The idea of bringing a child to the dentist to have his or her teeth cleaned twice a year is a false representation of what matters, he said—in fact, a futile effort. Dr. Barkley believed the most important service a professional practice can provide is effectiveness evaluation, support, encouragement, and coaching for *both* child and parents.

Is Our Stuff Interfering with Our Patients' Stuff?

How often do we find ourselves "mothering" our patients—especially if they have been in our practices for a long time? (We know that Mrs. Jones is going to have a hysterectomy, Ted's son just got arrested, and Mrs. Heel's cocker spaniel will be attending doggie discipline classes again, because Pooches failed the first time.) We know all kinds of "stuff" about our patients! In fact, their "stuff" sometimes causes us to feel bad when we describe the restorative care they need—and present the fees. But, what about *our* stuff?

Now, this may seem harsh, but too many discussions in the hygiene and treatment galleries are one-sided, with the slant towards the team instead of being centered on patient care. Please do not misunderstand me: Dental team members need to (and should) feel compassion and genuinely care for patients. But we cannot allow our patients' stuff, or our assumptions about their financial issues, to affect how (or if) we present our diagnostic findings and fees.

Perhaps you're not influenced by your patient's stuff. On the other hand, your personal "crossover points" may unconsciously control your clinical dialogue. Dr. Paul Homoly, author of PennWell's *Isn't It Wonderful When Patients Say "Yes"?* talks about the crossover points—those points at which treatment and/or fee discussions become so ominous that you hesitate to mention them. Your objectivity "crosses over" into fear of presenting fees, fear of the treatment, fear of creating an angry patient, fear of not knowing what to say when the patient asks, "Is the dentist buying a new car?," and/or fear of rejection.

Many times, we unconsciously allow our beliefs and our fears of our patients' reactions to the recommended dentistry—and the fees—to affect the treatment protocols that we present. For example: If your office charges $1,500 a crown, and if you believe that the fee is too high or unjustified (based on the dentist's clinical ability, knowledge, or skill), then you begin to place yourself in your patient's shoes. You assume that because *you* think $1,500 is a lot of money to pay for a crown, then your patients will feel the same way. You base this conclusion on the "stuff" that you think you know about your patients. So, rather than begin a conversation in which you have already decided the outcome, you—in your mind at least—decide not to offer the clinical findings and fees.

But what team members must realize, is this: Just because we may know a little about the patient's life, and just because *we* may not be able to afford the smile-design case, this does not mean that our patients cannot afford it. Team members must appreciate that *treatment is not about them*, but about their *patients*. It is not our responsibility to sugar-coat or place on hold any of our patients' oral-health concerns, because in doing so, we assume they are not ready to hear it, they cannot afford it. We have a legal, moral, and ethical responsibility to be oral-health experts, and that includes sharing the good and not-so-good news. So, after your next prediagnostic examination, don't be afraid to present an accurate assessment of the patient's needs, including an accurate estimate of costs involved. Say it loud and say it proud!

Create Your Strategies

The secret to success is to be ready when your opportunity comes.

• **Benjamin Disraeli**

This exercise, provided at the end of each chapter, will assist you in designing a game plan based on each chapter's topics to develop the skills, knowledge, and expertise necessary to propel you to your next level of personal and professional growth. Ask, answer, and record the following:

My professional goals for becoming an aesthetic detective in the future are:

_____

_____

_____

The areas for which I feel I need assistance and support to achieve my goals are:

_____

_____

_____

My action steps to get in the game and achieve those goals are:

_____

_____

_____

My list of specific goals and dates I wish to accomplish them includes:

_____

_____

_____

Possible obstacles to watch out for: (i.e., fear of rejection, fear of change, lack of accountability, denial, lack of focus, lack of self-evaluation, lack of mentoring relationships, etc.):

_____

_____

_____

Section II

Hygiene Potential

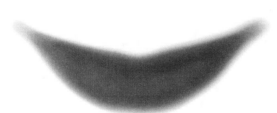

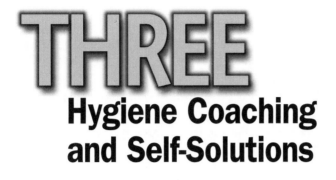

THREE
Hygiene Coaching and Self-Solutions

Giving never moves in a straight line, it always travels in circles.

• Robert Schuller

Reaching Concordance: A Better Way to "Comply"

By Jill Rethman, R.D.H., B.A.

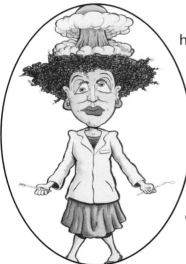

Fig. 3-1: *Hygienist burnout.*

It's Monday morning. Gladys Grungemouth has just entered your operatory for her recare appointment. You're thinking, "What a great way to start the week! Mrs. Grungemouth never listens to what I tell her about self-care, and she's so negative!" After the superficial pleasantries are exchanged, Mrs. Grungemouth sits in your chair. She's thinking, "What a great way to start the week! Helen Hygiene always yells at me for not flossing, and doesn't understand how difficult it is for me to do it. I wish she would just clean my teeth and leave me alone."

Sound familiar? (Fig. 3-1)

A common concern among dental professionals is patient motivation. We use our best professional skills to treat patients while they are in the operatory, but how they perform oral hygiene self-care procedures often determines whether or not they are periodontally healthy.

Self-care is especially important to patients with aesthetic restorations. Improper or inefficient care can render the most beautiful aesthetic procedures null and void. Therefore, along with the treatment we render, a large part of our dental hygiene role is to educate patients about appropriate self-care measures.

This educational process is two-fold, involving a review of procedures and recommendations to perform them as directed. The latter aspect has been traditionally called patient compliance. A new term—concordance—has recently been introduced in the medical literature. Following is a brief review of these terms and how they are used in contemporary dental hygiene care.

Compliance: Our world versus the real world

Our definition of compliance, as members of the healthcare field, is "the extent to which a person's behavior coincides with health-related advice." Such a definition connotes cooperation on the part of a patient to follow through with professional recommendations. However, if we review the term compliance from the patient's perspective, it is apparent that a discrepancy exists.

According to *Webster's Unabridged Dictionary*, compliance is "a yielding, as to a request, wish, desire, demand or proposal; a disposition to yield to others." This definition implies a concession or submission on the patient's part—not cooperation. Furthermore, if we examine synonyms for the term *non*compliance, we find the following words: "disobedience, resistance, rebelliousness, assertiveness, stubbornness, and obstinacy."

It is clear, then, that use of the term compliance creates confusion for clinicians and patients. Moreover, it defines two completely different ways to view self-care. The term—and, more important, the *mindset* of compliance—does not promote a feeling of teamwork. Instead, it conjures up a battle of wills.

Concordance: Reaching common ground

An important first step in motivation is to assure the patient, "We are on the same team and working together to achieve a common goal." The patient must know that the clinician is available to offer support, as needed. In addition, the patient needs to feel ownership of his or her condition and to remain a part of the decision-making process. Together, patient and clinician should reach an agreement as to the best approach to meet an individual's needs. This agreement can be termed *concordance*.

Concordance implies an open, honest discussion between clinician and patient. It requires that both reach a mutual understanding on the nature of an illness as well as the appropriate treatment. This notion is important. Commonly, a clinician may think that a patient would automatically accept recommendations because the clinician is a professional. Past experience shows, however, that this is not the case, since patient motivation is an ongoing concern in oral healthcare.

Let's go back to the Monday morning situation we discussed and look at it in another light.

It's Monday morning. Gladys Grungemouth has just entered your operatory for her recare appointment. You're thinking, "What a great way to start the week! I know I haven't been able to motivate Mrs. Grungemouth to floss as she should, and I'm really concerned about the gingival health around her new veneers. I'm going to try my best to identify how she can keep those areas healthy. Maybe I need to look at other options besides floss."

Working toward success: Together

With this concept in mind, you proceed to ask Mrs. Grungemouth how she has been doing with her oral hygiene. Instead of voicing your usual, "Have you been using your dental floss?" question, you say, "Show me how you use floss." When she proceeds to do so, it becomes obvious where and why she is having difficulty. You then tell Mrs. Grungemouth that this time, you'd like to work with her to try a new method. You show her intra-dental brushes, rubber tips, wooden sticks, or a new automated device. Ask her to pick which one she'd like to use for a trial period and tell her that you and she will re-evaluate the product at her next appointment.

Mrs. Grungemouth is thinking, "What a great way to start the week! Helen Hygiene always yells at me for not flossing, but now she understands how difficult it is for me to do it. I can't wait to try this new product and see if it works for me." You and Mrs. Grungemouth have just reached concordance.

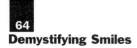

Conclusion

Concordance demands a mindset different than that of *compliance*. It requires continuing communication between patient and clinician. Most important, it obliges a team effort—not simply coercion or demands on the part of the clinician, more than obeying or yielding on the part of the patient. Since motivation has been a frustrating goal for many of us, let's change the way we view it. Start thinking concordance and not compliance.

Dry Brushing: Linguals First

by Trisha E. O'Hehir, R.D.H., B.S.

Rarely does a hygienist see mandibular anterior lingual surfaces with no calculus formation. For some of us, this is actually a periodontal screening tool. A quick look at the lower linguals and we have a pretty good idea of what awaits us. This quick check tells us if we can expect to stay on schedule or run late. Our time and skills are better spent providing other services rather than removing this deposit time after time. But how do we eliminate this problem?

Despite greater accumulation of both hard and soft deposits, and higher levels of bleeding on probing for mandibular lingual surfaces, standard toothbrushing focuses little or no time on this area. There is a very simple, inexpensive way to prevent the formation of supragingival calculus on the lingual surfaces of the lower anterior teeth. Just imagine: Your patients returning with no buildup on the lower lingual surfaces. (Fig. 3–2)

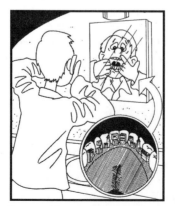

Fig. 3–2: *No build-up on the lower lingual surfaces.*
Courtesy of Trisha E. O'Hehir, R.D.H., B.S. All rights reserved.

The answer is not chemicals to inhibit calculus formation, but removal of the bacterial plaque before it *becomes* calculus. Sounds simple. But is it achievable? Yes—it is achievable, and it is very simple. Here's how it works: *Brushing the lower linguals first with a dry toothbrush.* It sounds too simple to actually work, but the results of this two-step process are amazing! Practical experience, as well as scientific research, confirms these findings. A pilot study of 129 private-practice patients across the United States demonstrated the effectiveness of this approach. Simply telling patients to dry brush the lingual surfaces first resulted in reductions of bleeding scores by 55 percent for all mandibular lingual surfaces. Calculus scores were reduced an average of 58 percent for all mandibular lingual surfaces—63 percent for the mandibular anterior section and 49 percent for the mandibular posterior section.

Many dental hygienists the world over have discovered, on their own, the benefits of dry brushing and brushing the linguals first. If the idea is new to you, test it yourself.

How does such a simple change in brushing work? Most people brush the "outsides" first and the "insides" last. Toothpaste use guarantees very little time for this area, as most people brush until the bubbles threaten to overtake them. That is the signal they use to determine how long to brush. When they are nearly drowning in bubbles, they give a quick swish of the brush over the linguals of the lower anteriors, just before they quit. (Fig. 3–3)

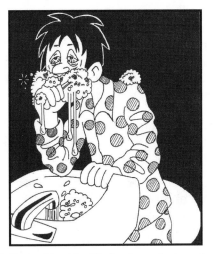

Fig. 3–3: A quick swish of the brush over the lower linguals.
Courtesy of Trisha E. O'Hehir, R.D.H., B.S. All rights reserved.

We traditionally hold our toothbrushes under running water before brushing, with or without toothpaste. That was necessary when all the toothbrushes were made of hard bristles, but the soft bristles we currently use do not need to be water-softened. Dry brushing first on the lower linguals utilizes the slight stiffness of dry bristles to mechanically remove bacterial plaque.

People tend to brush longer where they start—not where they finish. Starting on the lower linguals will give that area at least a fighting chance. Brushing dry assures that the bristles will be slightly stiffer and better able to remove sticky plaque. Simply changing the routine to start on the lingual of the lower anteriors will assure more plaque removal.

Aside from bristle stiffness, there are several other reasons why dry brushing removes bacterial plaque, and therefore, prevents the buildup of supragingival calculus. First, toothpaste bubbles prevent us from looking in the mirror as we brush. The tendency is to lean over the sink and drool and daydream, rather than think about specific areas to be brushed. This is necessary, since the bubbles would otherwise splatter the mirror and generally cause a mess of the person brushing, as well as the bathroom. Because of the bubbles and the daydreaming, it may seem that we have actually brushed for several minutes, when in fact, it may be little more than 30 seconds.

Strong flavoring in toothpaste may be the most critical factor. It can produce a false sense of effective plaque removal, leaving the tongue slightly numb, and leading one to think the mouth is clean and slippery, when there may actually be a great deal of plaque remaining. We are tricked into thinking the teeth are clean when in fact, they aren't. This may explain why so many patients who brush immediately before seeing the hygienist still have heavy plaque accumulations; they think their teeth are clean because they feel slippery. The strong flavor in the toothpaste has numbed their tongue.

Dry brushing allows people to look in the mirror and see where to put the brush. It also increases the length of time spent brushing. Achieving the goal of more thorough plaque removal requires more than 30 seconds' work. A brushing time of just 30 seconds allows for less than a single second of brushing in any one area. (This figure is calculated by estimating the number of brushing areas in the mouth to be 36.

If each brushing area includes only two to three teeth, that gives us eight brushing areas for each side of an arch—16 upper and 16 lower, plus four occlusal areas, for a total of 36 brushing areas.) To spend five seconds in each area requires a full three minutes of brushing evenly throughout the mouth. That usually doesn't happen.

Brushing first in areas that are prone to heavy deposits will result in greater reductions in plaque and calculus accumulation. After the plaque has been removed with the dry brush, a second brushing should be performed using toothpaste, for stain removal and to provide therapeutic fluoride as needed.

Home Irrigation with the Water Pik Oral Irrigator: The Most Effective Self-Care Device You're Not Recommending

by Carol Jahn, R.D.H., M.B.A.

A recent survey in *Dental Products Report* says that only 24 percent of dental offices recommend home irrigation to patients. This number is troubling because it means that almost three-quarters of practitioners are overlooking an important health care device with a proven scientific track record in significantly improving oral health.

Despite the fact that the research on home irrigation has always been positive, practitioner opinion has often waxed and waned. Most likely, this has been due to misconceptions perpetrated about irrigation. Like most myths, however, these notions are not based on reality. In fact, in almost every case, they are easily disputed by sound scientific evidence.

Here are the real facts on home irrigation as supported by the research.

Patients who use daily home water irrigation have been able to show statistically significant and clinical relevant reductions in:

- Gingivitis

- Bleeding on probing

- Periodontal pathogens

- Pro-inflammatory mediators

So, what does this mean for you, your patients, and their aesthetic restorations? Just this: The healthier the tissue, the better the aesthetic appearance. Because home irrigation reduces gingivitis and bleeding, your patients who use it can expect firm, healthy-looking tissue that does not bleed. From a cosmetic aspect, this will enhance the appearance of the aesthetic restoration and, in turn, your patient's happiness. Clinically, tight margins that are easy to clean can help increase the longevity of the restorations. In more than 40 studies conducted on home irrigation, the practice has been found to be safe for both hard and soft tissue as well as dental materials.

Do patients really need to add irrigation to their regimen if they are already brushing and flossing? Probably not, if your patient shows absolutely no bleeding anywhere. However, because most patients *do* suffer some areas of gingivitis or bleeding, adding home irrigation can go a long way to help eliminate residual inflammation. Many studies have demonstrated that adding home irrigation to a brushing and flossing routine enhances the reduction of gingivitis and bleeding by as much as 50 percent.

What solution should we recommend? We try to have our patients avoid any product that contains alcohol or that can cause staining. The good news about daily home irrigation is that water works! Rather than the basic mechanical action that we are accustomed to with tooth brushing and flossing, or even the pharmacotherapeutic action of some mouth rinses, irrigation is most effective subgingivally—disrupting and dispersing pathogens in the loosely attached plaque and reducing bone-destroying inflammatory agents in the gingival crevicular fluid. New, critical research on home irrigation has shown it has a modulating effect on pro-inflammatory agents in the gingival crevicular fluid. These agents are products of the body's host response that stimulate bleeding, attachment loss, and bone destruction. These findings mean that irrigation is probably less about the agent used and more about its overall effects on the immune response. (Fig. 3–4)

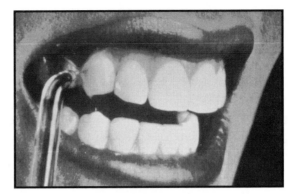

Fig. 3–4: *Effects of irrigation.*

How can I ask my patients to do one more thing? If your patient is not enjoying better oral health from the devices you are already recommending, it is time for a critical re-evaluation of what *is* working for your patient. As you do this, keep in mind this tongue-in-cheek definition of insanity: "Doing the same thing over and over again, and expecting a different result." Rather than just adding devices, it is important to collaborate with patients to find the products they are most open to using. How you frame the message or recommendation has a powerful impact on patient acceptance. Your enthusiasm is a powerful motivational tool, and honesty is the best policy.

A doctor once shared this interesting story about one of his patients and home irrigation. Many years ago, shortly after home irrigators first came on to the market, a dentist recommended home irrigation to one of his patients. The reply he received was a cold, "I'll think about it." A few months later, the patient returned for a maintenance visit. She requested that the doctor look at her *gums,* "and tell me if I still need that Waterpik." The doctor realized he was being challenged. He performed his exam, and at the conclusion, told his patient, "Your mouth has really improved. The tissue looks great. There is no bleeding. So honestly, no—you don't need to buy that Waterpik." The patient looked at him and broke out in a huge, warm smile. "Doctor" she said, "I bought it and started using it six months ago!" Forty years later, this doctor is still recommending the Waterpik oral cleaning system with great results and happy patients.

Isn't it time *you* started recommending home irrigation?

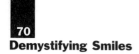

Fluoride Utilization in the 21st Century

by Tricia Osuna, R.D.H., B.S.
Sultan Chemists

Fluorides and their use for the prevention of dental caries have been highly researched and discussed for more than 50 years. Fluoride's unique affects on caries progression, as well as caries initiation, have been, at times, controversial among dental professionals and lay communities. Historically, the benefits of professional fluoride use through in-office gel/foam delivery, systemic delivery, and take-home products have been associated with the prevention of dental caries. However, the action of fluoride on plaque has important preventive as well as therapeutic benefits on periodontal infections and oral health maintenance.[1]

It is imperative for all dental professionals to understand the effectiveness of fluorides as caries prevention agents and to have knowledge of the protocols for utilization of all available fluoride products. Adherence to these protocols will ensure efficient and effective use of appropriate fluorides.

History of fluorides

Pioneering work in the 1940s found that it was generally believed that the major caries-preventive affect of fluoride was pre-eruptive.[2]

Recommendations were based on the assumption that incorporation of fluoride in the enamel apatite lattice would confer the enamel a resistance to acid dissolution, i.e., that a high intake of fluoride during tooth formation and mineralization would result in fluoride-rich enamel, with enduring resistance to dental caries.[3]

As research into the properties and effects of fluoride continued, it became apparent that a high concentration of fluoride in the hard dental tissues was of less importance than a moderate increase in fluoride concentration in oral fluids.[4]

Dean's research was accepted for approximately 25 years. At that time, fluoride's mode of action was thought to be its incorporation into the apatite-like crystals during development, resulting in crystals that were highly resistant to subsequent post-eruptive acid attack. However, when compared to its post-eruptive effects, the pre-eruptive mode of action is now considered to be very minor. Dental professionals currently accept fluoride mechanics as caries-preventive and caries-controlling in the post-eruptive phase as the standard for fluoride delivery to their patients.

Mode of action

Fluoride utilization is the second most effective method for prevention of dental caries. (Removal of debris is the first.) Modern concepts of fluoride mechanisms of action emphasize daily use to establish and maintain a significant concentration in saliva and plaque fluid, thereby maintaining a level of fluoride dissolution in the enamel surface. While the caries inhibition of fluoride has been proven to be almost totally post-eruptive, the pre-eruptive benefits are obvious during the developmental phase of tooth eruption, where occlusal pits and fissures are protected by fluoride utilization in the post-eruptive phase.

Fluoride is at its highest levels close to the surface, where the tissue contacts fluid that supplies the fluoride ion. Enamel surfaces, in the pre-eruptive stages, benefit from topical application, while the pulpal chamber releases fluoride that has been stored in the mineralized tissue from ingestion, via the dentinal layers.

When preparations containing a high content of fluoride are applied to the teeth, calcium fluoride precipitates out to provide free fluoride ions. Fluoride ions act as a reservoir of fluoride during demineralization and remineralization. The ions remain in solution until the pH drops below 6.0 in dental plaque during a cariogenic challenge. The ions then released can prevent demineralization by entering partially demineralized crystals and begin to remineralize them. Re-mineralized areas often have increased mineral content when compared with their previous state. The presence of fluoride ions greatly enhances remineralization.[5]

Patients who suffer from xerostomia, orthodontic patients, those who have highly cariogenic diets, or patients who have less than adequate oral hygiene routines are excellent candidates for fluoride treatments, as they are commonly regarded as high-caries-risk patients. Patients with low-caries risk also benefit from topical fluoride due to the ability of fluoride to reduce acid formation in the dental plaque, reduce plaque adhesion, and change the ecology of the plaque microflora, thereby preventing the formation of carious lesions. Caries can be prevented through mechanical removal of bacteria, but a program that combines fluoride therapy and improved oral hygiene maintenance is most beneficial for these particular patients.

Documented statistics show that 17 percent of pediatric patients account for 67 percent of the total caries experience.[6] These data should translate into foundational principles for clinical modalities that support specific analysis of exposures to fluoride and determination of the types of fluoride to be used during in-office procedures. Knowing the appropriate fluoride selection—acidulated phosphate fluoride (APF) or neutral sodium fluoride (NaF)—is key in treating specific patient needs and aiding their ability to comply with in-office treatment as well as adjunctive prescription (take-home) fluorides.

Topical fluoride utilization

APF was first introduced in the early 1960s. At that time, these agents contained 1.23 percent fluoride in the form of sodium fluoride at pH 3.0. Phosphate was added to an acid solution to depress calcium fluoride formation and increase fluorapatite formation.[7] APF has been used for caries inhibition as research has demonstrated enamel remineralization. The majority of fluoride uptake into enamel using a 1.23 percent APF gel has been proven to occur during the first minute of application. During the next three minutes of application, additional uptake occurs. Nonetheless, there appear to be several advantages to using the one-minute application procedure for APF instead of the four-minute application.

The one-minute procedure:

• Lessens the potential for fluoride ingestion

• Decreases the adverse effects of etching of aesthetic restorations

• Increases patient tolerance

• Improves patient acceptance

A patient classified as an active caries risk would require APF fluoride applications of 1.23 percent twice a year; a patient with rampant caries should receive topical fluoride treatments on a quarterly basis and may also require a home fluoride treatment program to control caries formation.[8]

Sodium fluoride gel

Neutral Sodium Fluoride (NaF) was first introduced in the early 1940s as a 0.1 percent aquaeous solution to be applied at four-month internals for two years. Currently NaF is applied in a 2 percent gel and is recommended for patients with root caries, Xerostomia, orthodontic appliances, and aesthetic restorations (laminate veneers, porcelain or composite restorations).

While very effective, sodium fluoride is recommended for four-minute delivery only. It has been clinically proven to reduce caries and is most beneficial to patients when delivered at three-month intervals accompanied by prescription fluoride for take-home usage.

Clinical application

Topical agents are safe and considered harmless, but must be used as directed by the manufacturer. When administering fluoride through a tray method for children less than 16 years of age, certain procedures should be followed to minimize ingestion of the gel/foam. Recommendations include:

- Limiting the amount of gel/foam to no more than 2 ml or 40 percent of the tray capacity
- Limiting gel to 5 to 10 drops in the tray
- Using a timer
- Seating the patient in upright position with head tilted forward
- Using suction throughout the fluoride treatment
- Continuing to use suction for 30 seconds after application and/or expectorate saliva for approximately one minute
- Never leaving a child unattended while administering a fluoride treatment
- Keeping fluoride solutions out of reach of a pediatric patient

In-office delivery of fluoride is best when administered with a tray specifically designed for this purpose. On rare occasions, cotton rolls and swabs may be used instead of a fluoride delivery tray. Fluoride delivery using a tray method consists of these steps:

- Select tray of appropriate size

- Entire dentition must be covered, including areas of recession, while allowing for gel to come in contact with the tooth structure

- Ends of tray (distal portion) should be closed to ensure that gel does not flow over into patient's mouth

- Foam-lined trays are ideal, as they conform to patients' dentition and allow for flow of gel to all surfaces

- Place gel in tray as described above

- Insert tray into patient's mouth

- Insert saliva ejector between trays, being sure that patient is comfortable. Cotton rolls may need to be used on opposite quadrants to balance occlusion with this method

- Remove tray from patient's mouth

- Advise patient to expectorate immediately following tray removal

- Utilize high-volume suction, if necessary, to remove excess fluoride following treatment

- Advise patient not to eat or drink for 30 minutes following procedure

Use of home fluoride

Use of prescription home fluorides benefits patients with individualized needs such as decalcification, which often accompanies orthodontic treatment; dentinal hypersensitivity; root caries; post-periodontal surgery; recurrent decay; xerostomia, and/or post head-and-neck radiation therapy. Two types of home fluorides—stannous 0.4 percent and sodium 1.1 percent fluoride gels or pastes—are recommended.

Stannous fluoride 0.4 percent gel is recommended for patients with dentinal hypersensitivity, as it occludes the dentinal tubules, inhibits plaque accumulation, and protects areas at risk for decalcification. When prescribing stannous fluorides, the professional must take into consideration prior dental restorative treatment, because the product may cause extrinsic stains on aesthetic restorations, as well as natural dentition.

Stannous fluoride is most beneficial to patients when used at least once per day and allowed to remain on dentinal surfaces for one minute while brushing. Remind the patient to swish fluoride for one minute and then expectorate following tooth brushing. This recommendation will benefit your patient because it allows the fluoride ion to penetrate the tooth structure.

Sodium fluoride 1.1 percent take-home gel is routinely prescribed for patients with aesthetic restorations who need more protection for caries reduction, especially patients with a history of cervical caries, patients suffering from xerostomia, or after head-and-neck radiation therapy when patients cannot tolerate an acidic environment. Sodium fluoride pastes/gels sweetened with Xylitol provide an additional benefit to patients in light of recent research on Xylitol and plaque inhibition. Sodium fluoride is ideal for patients suffering from sensitivity due to the use of whitening agents. Fluorides with lower concentrations provide a reduced dose of fluoride, which replenishes fluoride in the tooth structure, saliva, and plaque and supports the mineralization process for all individuals regardless of their caries risk assessment.

Take-home applications are recommended following a regular brushing or as a daily dentifrice. Optimal results occur when patients expectorate and do not rinse for at least 30 minutes after use.[9]

Conclusion

Fluoride therapy is considered an important modality for the prevention of decay; to aid in the remineralization of incipient lesions; to reduce dentinal hypersensitivity, and to reduce plaque accumulation. Fluorides offer additional benefits to dental patients in many areas, such as oral hygiene instruction, nutritional counseling, and comprehensive restorative and diagnostic treatment plans. In addition, customized fluoride modalities may provide optimal care.

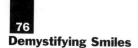

Complementary and Alternative Medicine

Adapted with permission from lecture handouts and personal notes,
Complementary and Alternative Medicine: The Role of the Dental Professional,
presented by Leslie Andrews, R.D.H., M.B.A. Supported through an educational grant from Philips Oral Healthcare, makers of Sonicare.

Complementary and alternative medicine (CAM) represents varied healing philosophies and therapies that conventional, mainstream medicine often disregards. Most people understand CAM to be the use of modalities such as acupuncture, herbs, homeopathy, therapeutic massage, and traditional oriental medicines to treat health conditions and maintain well-being.

CAM treatments and therapies may be used singularly, as an alternative to conventional therapies, or alongside conventional, mainstream therapies, in a complementary, integrative approach. CAM therapies are often referred to as holistic, meaning they take into account "the whole person" and not just the ailment they seek to treat.

CAM's growing popularity in the United States

The United States Congress established the National Center for Complementary and Alternative Medicine (NCCAM) in 1998, allied with the National Institutes of Health (NIH). The goal was "to stimulate, develop, and support research on CAM for the benefit of the public," according to the NCCAM charter. The underlying philosophy of NCCAM is to be "an advocate for quality science, rigorous and relevant research, and open and objective inquiry into which CAM practices work, which do not, and why."

NCCAM surveys report that 33 percent of Americans used an alternative therapy in 1990, rising to more than 42 percent in 1997. Therapies most often were reported to be herbal medicine, massage, megavitamins, self-help groups, folk remedies, energy healing, and homeopathy. In addition, NCCAM reports that Americans spent more than $27 billion on these therapies in 1997, "exceeding out-of-pocket spending for all U.S. hospitalizations."

A NCCAM-cited survey, first published in 1994, claims that "more than 60 percent of doctors from a wide range of specialties recommended alternative therapies to their patients at least once. In addition, 47 percent of the doctors in this study reported using alternative therapies themselves." In 1998, 75 of 117 United States medical schools surveyed offered elective courses in CAM "or included CAM topics in required courses." Still another survey found that people turn to CAM remedies both because they are dissatisfied with "conventional medicine" and because "these health care alternatives mirror their own values, beliefs, and philosophical orientations toward health and life."

So, dental professionals integrating alternative therapies into their practices are encouraged to investigate CAM and how they may lead to positive clinical outcomes for their patients.

Develop strategies for—

- Educating yourself and your patients regarding this emerging and popular field

- Increasing your understanding of therapies, products, herbs, and supplements

- Promoting dialog between your patient and all of their health/oral health providers.

Areas to consider:

Homeopathy. CAM profession with therapeutic products

Naturopathy. CAM profession with a wide variety of therapies and products

Acupuncture. CAM profession with specific therapies

Traditional Chinese medicine. Discipline under which acupuncture falls (includes Chinese herbs)

Reflexology. Form of massage

Ayurvedic. System of wellness

Meditation. Relaxation technique

Yoga. A discipline

Hypnosis. A technique using a machine

Chiropractic. CAM profession with specific therapies

Osteopathy. Conventional profession with specific therapies

Holistic or biological dentistry. Not recognized by the ADA

Self-Care Continuum

Pre-smile enrollment evaluations and subsequent post-restorative hygiene management sessions should dedicate an appropriate amount of focus to the what, why, how, and how much of oral self-care products.

Since proper care of restorative dentistry depends on the combined efforts of the oral health team and the patient, these pre-smile-design hygiene appointments present an opportunity for the dental hygienist to document and discuss the patient's current self-care. Establishing a clear and precise understanding of current product use is the first step in educating and creating a self-care program that is in alignment with their new smile.

Possible areas that should be covered include the use of:

- brushes (manual/power)
- polishes/pastes
- interproximal "smile cleaning" devices
- rinses
- tongue gels or sprays
- tongue deplaquers
- fluorides
- power irrigation devices
- fresh breath products (gum, sprays, mints, etc.)

The patient must be proficient in maintaining healthy gingival tissue, with emphasis placed on the importance of daily plaque elimination. These goals must be achieved without causing harm to the dentistry or soft tissue. Pre-smile demonstrations may begin with smile-brushing methods. Improper brushing techniques—scrubbing, excessive speed or pressure, and/or ineffective plaque removal—may affect the longevity of the aesthetic restorations and irritate gingival margins.

Based on current research, clinicians can extrapolate and recommend the modified Bass technique using a frequently changed soft-bristle toothbrush as the fundamental part of a self-care plan. Meticulous and proper oral hygiene behaviors can also be achieved though the use of a power toothbrush and low-abrasive toothpaste. A post-treatment demonstration may involve ensuring that the patient can remove interproximal bacteria without the aid catching or getting stuck between the dentistry. How often a patient uses a smile brush— what toothpaste or smile rinse, etc.—gives the dental hygienist clear insights into the possibility of the patient over-cleaning or using a product that may lead to aggressive applications or a preoccupation with his or her smile. This information, when recorded, may help derail potential gingival recession, restoration abrasion, and/or excessive patient cleaning.

Crystallizing why patients use certain products often provides a better understanding of who they listen to concerning their oral health care. Did the product recommendation originate from one of your practice's team members, a previous dental hygienist, a neighbor, the sales clerk—or Vanna White, via a television infomercial?

Thoroughly and legibly documenting all answers (option: computerized forms and charts) allows a seamless consistency of care among providers within one practice. If details from the first self-care conversation are written or recorded in their entirety, the clinical provider at the next session can easily continue the educational process without asking the same questions again. When patients see several providers, it is important that they have the perception that the previous dental hygienist valued the discussion enough to record it and that the current hygienist took the time to audit the chart and become familiar with the patient's oral health wants and self-care history.

With the initial information acquired, the hygienist may need to recommend changes to the routine. Beyond proper self-care practices, new smile product recommendations may need to be covered—including how many times a day the product should be effectively implemented and why the recommendation is being made.

Continuing care plans and interventions should be arranged based on the nature of aesthetic treatments and individual needs. Supportive aesthetic therapies (see chapter 5) can be incorporated into the standardized recare appointment. In a majority of cases, however, *aesthetic/restorative management sessions* should be included in the hygiene treatment plan. This change in terminology or description—from recare or maintenance visit to the aesthetic/restorative management session—emphasizes preserving the patient's dental investment. Whether the services performed at such appointments fall under the umbrella of supportive aesthetic care or supportive periodontal care— even a combination of the two—the patient needs to understand that it is "not just a cleaning." Patients *must* value the necessity of such appointments, and it needs to be communicated during case presentations. Fees, the proposed schedule, the length of appointment times, and the services to be provided all need to be communicated to the patient and incorporated into the restorative treatment and total financial plan.

Over-the-counter toothpastes

Consumer interest in smile-enhancing procedures is evident by the billion-dollar over-the-counter market for products that whiten and brighten teeth. However, the mass marketing of over-the-counter (OTC) oral-health products confuses our patients; in fact, they are *so* confused, they will trust their oral health to celebrities selling products via infomercials or informational print advertisements! Oral health professionals need to understand the indications and limitations of dentifrices and educate their patients in choosing the appropriate partner for smile enhancement and/or aesthetic treatment preservation.

Let's take a moment to review the makeup of dentifrices. Traditionally, they have active and inactive ingredients. Active ingredients perform a specific preventive or treatment action. Some examples may include chlorine dioxide, essential oils, zinc chloride, fluoride, peroxides, potassium nitrate, and zinc compounds. Inactive ingredients include cleansing agents, humectants, color, preservative, sweeteners, flavors, foaming agents, thickening agents, and/or buffering agents. They provide structure, texture, color, flavor, stability, and cleaning activity.

Now, put yourself into the minds of your patients. They look into the mirror and smile. What do they see? Some may see their teeth getting darker close to their gingival line. Others see natural teeth turning yellow or exhibiting a blue-gray tone. They may also observe teeth that are discolored due to age, smoking, a diet filled with dark-pigmented foods and beverages, or other behavioral factors. Many patients see these darker areas and begin to self-treat with whitening toothpaste.

Clinicians may determine that the darker areas are exposed cementum or dentin, or the darkening may be a combination of extrinsic and intrinsic stain. Extrinsic stain can be yellow, green, orange, brown, and/or black. It could also be undetected decay or calculus. Internal stain may be blue-gray or yellow, probably caused by chemicals or systemic medications during tooth development, and impregnated deep within the dentin. Oral health teams can develop and implement a care plan that includes an appropriate dentifrice to benefit patients' individual oral status and smile.

Whitening toothpastes utilize four mechanisms in their attempt to change the color of teeth. These include abrasion, chemical dissolution, peroxide lightening, and cosmetic masking. Dentifrices usually contain a mixture of cleansing agents (silicas 20 to 40 percent) to ensure efficient cleaning. Some abrasives *do* remove mild surface stains; however, the natural color of the dentition remains unchanged. Whitening is achieved by removing extrinsic stain and the results of abusive habits, which can lead to possible loss of tooth structure. This treatment, in other words—popular with the uninformed consumer—achieves questionable results at the expense of the enamel or dentin.

Chemicals have also been incorporated into dentifrices to enhance cosmetics. This treatment works twofold. The first is by the chemical dissolution of the stains from the tooth surface. Secondly, crystal growth inhibitors (tetrasodium pyrophosphate, disodium dihydrogen pyrophosphate, and sodium tripolyphosphate) limit plaque mineralization, which in turn prevents the growth of supragingival calculus. Many tartar control toothpastes use this process as the foundation of their effectiveness. The theory is that if enamel surfaces remain calculus free, the whitening effect is accomplished through the management of a clean supragingival surface. Again, this method does not change the natural shades of the teeth. Some patients using a dentifrice employing this method of whitening may experience temperature sensitivity to toothpastes whose chemicals are absorbed into the enamel or exposed dentin.

The benefit of peroxide as an oxidation agent has been well documented in dental literature. Peroxide-containing toothpastes are marketed to have the same results as professional, peroxide-containing whitening systems. However, let's reconsider the oxidation process. It occurs when oxygen combines with stain molecules in enamel and dentin to make organic stains more soluble. The resulting oxidation penetrates both enamel and dentin to remove organic material within the tubular structures and is dissolved into the saliva and oral environment. Carbamide peroxide and hydrogen peroxide are the most common active ingredients utilized in vital tooth whitening. Carbamide peroxide's contact time in a whitening tray can range from two to four hours and hydrogen peroxide's wear time is about 30 minutes. Ask yourself this: When was the last time one of your patients brushed their teeth for four hours?

Additional challenges found with these products are low concentrations (1 to 2 percent) of the peroxide and the immediate contamination of the toothpaste by bacteria and saliva.

The last option in the dentifrice category is cosmetic masking. Cosmetic dentifrices mask extrinsic stains with chemical compounds like titanium dioxide, a common ingredient in paint. Stains are not removed, but are theoretically covered with a lighter-colored material. The results of this option vary and are difficult to maintain.

The dentifrice story—how they affect natural dentitions—is further complicated by their effects on dental material systems. A majority of the research in this area has been performed *in vitro* and with varying research modalities and testing conditions. However, analyzing the information may prove to have some clinical significance. Keep in mind that the perfect dentifrice for aesthetic therapies and or ingredients has yet to be agreed upon.

Toothpaste and abrasion

Most studies in this area are conducted to compare the rate of abrasive wear and change in surface roughness of composite restorations when subjected to toothbrush-dentifrice abrasion. Ideally, a restoration should have an abrasion-resistance rate similar to that of enamel. Here are some summary points to guide you when choosing a dentifrice for your cosmetic patients:

- If the curing light is unable to completely cure the composite material (the ability of the wave length and intensity to ensure complete curing of photo initiators), this may decrease composite abrasion resistance.

- Unfilled resins (such as sealants) may exhibit higher wear rates and marginal leaking.

- Products with a low pH may show evidence of increased erosive/abrasive effects.

During your interactive patient examination, discuss frequency of brushing and technique. To ensure that the restorations are not being aggressively cared for, suggest brushing effectively (yet gently) three times a day with a low-abrasive tooth polish or paste. An overly aggressive toothpaste/toothbrush combination may adversely affect the aesthetic longevity, so educating about the dentifrice/ toothbrush combination is vital. The amount of toothpaste used each day, the length of time spent brushing, the pressure used, and any tooth sensitivity or gingival burning or sloughing should also be recorded in the patient's chart. Provide patients with both verbal and written instructions and product recommendations. The patient should be given a well-drafted and easy-to-follow guide as to where to get the recommended dentifrice and why the dental team is recommending this particular product. Lastly, the practitioner needs to reinforce to the patient that results are best maintained through professional supervision and excellent hygiene practices.

Aesthetic and restorative procedures are most successfully performed in a well-controlled environment, and they also provide clinicians the opportunity to educate that patient on how optimal oral hygiene is key in maintaining aesthetic results. Because many extrinsic stains are associated with the staining of dental plaque or the acquired pellicle, patients' self-care guidelines must include behavior modification with emphasis on effectively removing plaque and bacteria from the teeth surfaces and cosmetic treatments.

If patients choose to use a whitening dentifrice, remember to thoroughly explain to them the hypotheses behind whitening dentifrices. Tooth/restoration surfaces remain stain- and calculus-free from commitment to meticulous oral hygiene—not a special product!

Power brushes and gingival abrasion

When discussing and recommending appropriate self-care products, some patients may reveal the perception and/or experience that power brushes can cause gingival abrasion. This concern needs to be identified and addressed during self-care education. The reality, in nine out of 10 cases, is that no one ever took the time to teach them *how* to properly use the recommended power device.

This means that if you recommend a certain toothbrush for the patient's oral health, it is your responsibility to make sure the patient is properly instructed on how to use it.

Have you ever purchased a major appliance, taken it home, pulled out the instructions, and proceeded to try and put it together? (Does the word "frustration" come to mind?) The next time you made such a purchase, did you pay the extra charge to have it assembled and perhaps even delivered?

Similarly, this is how our patients sometimes feel. We send them out to buy a power brush or a product. When they get home, they may (but, probably more accurately, will not) read the directions before they attempt to put the product together, charge it, and use it. Ever wonder why long-term commitment to self-care products can be dismal?

Take time for the added value gained by educating patients on the products you recommend. Provide a self-care area in your office where personnel (like service personnel at department store cosmetic counters) provide demonstrations as part of your non-surgical periodontal program. You might add an additional charge for self-care instruction. Do *not* send your patients into the stores to fail! Establish a plan to manage or improve their oral health. Become a product coach.

Home service products: A dialogue

Here's an example of how you can verbally (or in writing—longhand or electronically) assist your patients in creating a dialogue and a strategy for educating them on the merits (versus hype!) of some self-care products.

Do you brush your smile/all your teeth every day?

- Manual or power?
- How many times a day?
- Product(s) used?
- Why did you choose that product(s)?

Do you clean between all your teeth every day?

- Clean between how?
- Manual or power?
- How many times a day?
- Product(s) used?
- Why did you choose that product(s)?

Do you use smile polish/ toothpaste everyday?

- How many times a day?
- Product(s) used?
- Why did you choose that product(s)?

Do you use a tongue cleaner everyday?

- Manual or power?
- How many times a day?
- Product(s) used?
- Why did you choose that product(s)?

Do you use a tongue spray/gel everyday?

- Manual or power?
- How many times a day?
- Product(s) used?
- Why did you choose that product(s)?

Do you use fluoride everyday?

- Rinse or gel?
- With or without tray?
- How many times a day?
- Product(s) used?
- Why did you choose that product(s)?

Do you use a water-powered cleaning/irrigator device everyday?

- Solution used?

- How many times a day?
- Product(s) used?
- Why did you choose that product(s)?

Do you or have you used a professionally dispensed whitening product?

- Type/system?
- In office, at home with trays, both, other?
- How many regimens?
- Times a day, week, and month?
- How often do you rewhiten? or use a touch-up?
- Why?
- Product(s) used?
- Why did you choose that product(s)/system?

Do you use an over-the-counter bleaching product/tooth-paste?

- Type
- Rinse, guards, strips, other?
- How many regimens?
- Times a day, week, and month?
- How often do you rewhiten? or use a touch-up?
- Why?
- Product(s) used?
- Why did you choose that product(s)/system?

Do you use fresh-breath products? (Gum, mints, candies, spray, gels)

- How many times a day?
- Sugar-free?
- Alcohol-free?

Home-service education: Summary tips

- Hygiene sessions prior to beginning the restorative phase, during the provisional stage, and post-operatively should be times to discuss patient self-care regimens and self-care products.

- The patient must be proficient in maintaining healthy gingival tissue, with emphasis placed on the importance of daily plaque elimination and commitment to recare management schedules.

- Improper brushing techniques—such as scrubbing, excessive speed, or pressure—and use of an inappropriate toothbrush may damage or wear tooth-colored restorations and irritate gingival margins. Since recent clinical studies show that premium quality power tooth brushing is "better than manual" brushing (while not causing increased gingival abrasion), it is suitable to recommend a power brush. Powered toothbrushes can conveniently eliminate any challenges with improper brushing techniques and/or dexterity, while ultimately securing health through effective plaque and stain removal and respecting the restorative systems.

- Published data are inconclusive as to which toothpastes can abrade the surface of aesthetic restorations. If it merits any clinical relevance, a low-abrasive "no frills" tooth polish should be recommended for self-care.

- Instructions to patients should include a demonstration of interproximal plaque/bacteria removal.

- The limited published studies addressing the effect of alcohol on tooth-colored restorations conclude that alcohol may affect the longevity of the restoration by softening the composite matrix, causing the possibility for increased staining and early breakdown. Patients are encouraged to dilute alcohol-containing rinses or switch to alcohol-free alternatives.

- In addition, conversations can support daily tongue deplaquing, sugar-free, fresh-breath-related products, and tobacco cessation as they can affect the total body and health of the periodontium.

- Bruxism, fingernail biting, chewing on pens, etc., can damage or dislodge restorations, as well as natural teeth. An evaluation for a nightgaurd may be appropriate, depending upon the treatment and past occlusion/TMD history

Is It Toothbrush Abrasion or the Paste Connection?

Rightly so, we have been recommending that our patients use a soft-bristle toothbrush to guard against any unnecessary gingival abrasion and loss of tooth structure during brushing. And we realize that abrasion—non-caries cervical lesions—have a multifactor etiology.

A strategy that may be worth further investigation is the toothpaste/toothbrush connection. That is: Incorrect brushing may not be totally at fault. Neither may a heavy-handed brusher or even a hard toothbrush. The problem may also have to do with the abrasiveness of the toothpaste.

Some research provides evidence that toothpaste may be retained in soft bristle toothbrushes. In addition, since the soft filaments are usually smaller and more flexible, they increase the contact area of the toothpaste.

Evaluate your patients' toothpastes to determine what best suits their needs, while being the least abrasive. And educate the patient to thoroughly rinse out the toothbrush between brushings.

Points to Consider When Making Recommendations

Courtesy of *Power Brushes: The New Standard*
(Braun- Oral-B Laboratories)

- Will the product improve your patient's oral health?

- Have you personally tried the product?

- Are there multiple brushhead options to fit every need?

- Does the product have a good guarantee?

- Is the product backed by solid clinical research?
- Will your patients use the product?
- How will you implement this in your practice?

Teaching Your Patient

- Give in-office instructions to patients
- Have a demo brush or the patient's brush available
- Ensure that office staff is trained to use the brush
- Provide ample time for instruction

Got Evidence-Based Research?

"Evidence based:" What is it?

Dentistry and dental hygiene are art as well as science. Each professional body of knowledge should grow from providing empirical models for care based upon a systematic review of the scientific literature, clinical trials, and research, plus clinical experience. Below are a few challenges that can block the rise in practicing evidence-based dentistry and dental hygiene.

- The practitioners themselves. Many are unwilling or unable to break away from traditional approaches they might have learned in school or were taught by a previous employer.

- Some continuing education lecturers fail to provide scientifically unbiased information to the listeners. At any continuing education venue, be the complete consumer of impartial information and demand full disclosure by the presenters.

- Some dental publications are not refereed journals. This means that when an article is submitted for publication, professionals with the knowledge in the subject do not review or validate the information. As a reader, do not hesitate to ask the author to provide references to support the content of the material.

- Many professionals rely solely on sales representatives for information they use to make treatment decisions. Manufacturers are great resources, but it is a good guideline to verify the manufacturers' claims with independent studies.

As clinicians, we must remain aware and learn about evidence-supported advances so that we can implement these techniques and treatment modalities into our daily practice.

"Research Affects Me? How?" Clinical Strategy

All of us are consumers; all of us are inundated with commercially available dentifrices that claim to whiten, brighten, fight malodor and gingivitis, and on and on. But as professionals, we must evaluate the research and make sure that the products compared in the study are in the same *category.* Make sure the research is not comparing apples to oranges! This is how we can best serve our patients.

For example: If a study compared the effectiveness of stain removal by manual brushing to the effectiveness of stain removal by power brushing—who would come out on top? Obviously, the power brush. Does that mean manual brushing is inferior? No. The research compared apples to oranges. For validation, the research should compare manual brushes to manual brushes and power brushes to power brushes.

The same applies to toothpaste. If a manufacturer claims that their advanced whitening, calculus-inhibiting product removes "statistically" more extrinsic stain when compared to another manufacturer's product—well, that is *not* really news! Anecdotally, we can determine that the product that has added stain-removing ingredients (tetra-sodium pyrophosphate, sodium bicarbonate, tripolyphosphate, peroxide, etc.) would remove more extrinsic stains than a product that did not incorporate those chemicals. But if we were shown the research that compares the top products that claim stain-removal capabilities, as well as the abrasive effect of theses toothpastes on the tooth structure—now, *that* would be worth reading!

Create Your Strategies

There can be no happiness if the things we believe in are different from the things we do. • **Freya Stark**

This exercise, provided at the end of each chapter, will assist you in designing a game plan to develop the skills, knowledge, and expertise necessary to propel you to your next level of personal and professional growth. Ask, answer, and record the following:

My self-care coaching goals for the future are:

_____

_____

_____

The areas for which I would like assistance and support to achieve my goals are:

_____

_____

_____

My action steps to get in the game and achieve those goals includes:

_____

_____

_____

My list of specific goals and dates I wish to accomplish them are:

_____

_____

_____

Possible obstacles to watch out for (*i.e.,* fear of rejection, fear of change, and lack of accountability, denial, lack of focus, lack of self-evaluation, lack of mentoring relationships):

_____

_____

_____

Notes

1. Wilkins, Esther M., Clinical Practice of the Dental Hygienist, Esther M. Wiliness, 8th ed. (1999)

2. Dean, H.T., Arnold, F.A., Jr. Elove, E. (1942) "Domestic water and dental caries V: Additional studies of the relation of fluoride domestic waters to dental caries experience in 4,425 white children aged 12-14 years in 13 cities in 4 states." Public Health Reports 57:1155-1179 (1942)

3. Axellson, P., "An introduction to risk prediction and preventive dentistry," 1:77-97 2000

4. Ogaard, B., Rolla, G., Dijkman, T., Ruben, J., Arends, Jet, "Effect of fluoride mouth rinsing on caries lesions in development of shark enamel: An in-situ model study" Scandinavian Journal of Dent Restorations, 99:372-377 (1991)

5. Wilkins, ibid.

6. Hicks, M.J., Flaitz, C.M., "Epidemiology of dental caries in the pediatric and adolescent population: a review of past and current trends Journal of Clinical Pediatric Dentistry 18:43-50 (1993)

7. Ogaard, B., Seppa, L., Rolla, G. "Professional Topical Fluoride Applications: Clinical Efficacy and Mechanism of Action," Advanced Dental Restorations 8(2): 190-201 (July 1994)

8. Garcia-Godoy, F., Hicks, M. J., Flaitz, C., Berg, J., "Acidulated phosphate fluoride treatment and formation of caries-like lesions in enamel: Effect of application time," Journal of Clinical Pediatric Dentistry 19: 2 (1995)

9. Ibid

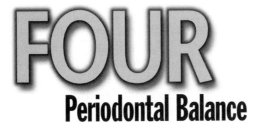

FOUR
Periodontal Balance

Everything we do is a process, and every process can be improved.
• **Ron Cristofano**

Advanced Clinical Thinking and Skills

If you were graduated from hygiene training more than 10 years ago, you'll remember being taught that calculus removal was the primary goal when cleaning someone's teeth. Some of us even had to mold a tooth out of wax and create it in an anatomically correct shape and then complete the project with a rub-down with nylons to make sure the mock-up tooth was smooth—*"just like the roots should be in our patient's mouth."* It was taught that hand instrumentation was the main means of mechanical root planing and that the primary goal of treatment was to remove the endotoxins that embedded themselves into the cementum of teeth. It was believed that to achieve acceptable results, all diseased cementum needed to be removed and an attempt made to remove all contaminated tooth structure.

Currently, even our regional board examiners prescribe to these limiting beliefs and measure a hygienist on the ability to "remove detectable calculus." But how relevant is that measure to our clinical practices of today?

There's never been a more exciting time to be a practicing hygienist. Hygienists are developing and providing a mastery of services in the many roles of healthcare providers, preventive specialists, periodontal co-therapists, aesthetic hygienists, and business partners. In addition, hygienists-as-preventive-specialists are also re-defining and centering their treatment on the whole client, with regard to disease prevention, health promotion, and guiding and supporting patients on the restorative care they need and the cosmetic care they desire. They're becoming better at understanding and contributing to the overall success of the practice by educating patients about the highest attainable periodontal health and restorative and esthetic possibilities. Add technologies to the mix, and future pacing your hygiene treatments, and the fun and learning never end!

The dental hygiene process of care (assessment, diagnosis, planing, implementation, and evaluation) must include all relevant, realistic, and evidence-based research findings and investigations supporting periodontal disease and restorative therapies. Make sure you are up to speed on these ever-changing modifiers to periodontal health:

- Oral disease and disorders affecting health and well-being throughout life (oral lesions, candidacies, birth defects, chronic facial pain, oral cancers)

- Safe and effective measures to prevent dental caries and periodontal disease, lifestyle behaviors that affect general health, and the effect on oral and craniofacicial health (tobacco/ smoking, excessive alcohol use, poor diet, stress, chewing or grinding teeth, etc.)

- How the mouth reflects the general health and well-being of the body ("mouth as a portal of entry"), and how oral disease and conditions are associated with other heath problems (genetics, diabetes, cardiovascular disease, stroke, pregnancy outcomes, puberty, medications)

Basic hygiene therapy

Therapeutic periodontal debridement is a basis of dental hygiene care. The goals are to arrest infection, remove plaque and calculus, reduce the amount of bioburden within the pocket, and provide an environment in which the tissue can return to health. A hygienist, after assessing the patient's health, can develop treatment modalities and select appropriate instruments to achieve the best clinical outcome.

Newer graduates have been versed in the growing information that shows complete cementum removal is not necessary to achieve a positive result. The debridement outcome has shifted to investigating the reduction of bioburden/microfilm within the periodontal pocket. Sonic and ultrasonic scalers are becoming the "must have" in clinical hygiene practices because they create a cavitation action when water or a chemotherapeutic agent hits the tips. This lavage helps in the reduction of bioburden within the pockets and facilitates healing.

Periodontal debridement's foundation is "cemented" in research that explains how bacterial plaque produces a bioburden that can be located supraginvially and subgingivally. The subgingival plaque fall into two categories—*adherent* and *non-adherent*. Adherent subgingival plaque and supragingival plaque mainly are comprised of gram-positive rods and cocci. However, the more virulent, non-adherent plaque (or tissue-associated plaque) makes up both gram-positive and gram-negative bacteria. When the non-adherent plaque infiltrates the periodontal tissues, a cascade of events and host immune response occurs. If not properly managed and treated, breakdown and destruction of the gingival, junctional epithelium, and bone may occur. Acknowledging that plaque is not the only cause of periodontal pathogenesis, however, debridement procedures must primarily focus on this factor.

Advances in non-surgical periodontal therapy are again shifting focus to the risks of recolonization of already-treated periodontal pockets and the effects on long-term periodontal stability. Repopulation or recontamination studies reveal that bacteria are transformed from one site to another, from one tooth to tooth another, or can spread from one person to another. Early-intervention clinical methods (*i.e.,* localized delivery of chemotherapeutic or antimicrobial agents that eliminate or drastically reduce the bioburden count in individualized pockets) have become the basis of future-focus debridement treatment strategies.

Often, when I speak with hygienists about restorative dentistry, hygienists wish their doctors would "go learn how to do some of the newer restorative treatments." The hygienist feels that the dentist's clinical skills need to be polished since his/her graduation. Well, let's look in the mirror, hygienist! How many hands-on clinical courses have *you* enrolled in since you were graduated? There are advances in ultrasonic instrumentation, local delivery anti-microbial products, lasers, local anesthetics, material management, and so on.

Fast-Tracking the Aesthetic and Restorative Treatment Plan via Full-Mouth Disinfection

by Kristy Menage Bernie, R.D.H., B.S.

The ultimate challenge in maximizing aesthetic and restorative treatment plan is to assure optimal oral health. Optimal oral health includes absence of disease, and, in this case, periodontal infection in particular can undermine the most innovative dental treatment plan. Aesthetics represent an opportunity to appeal to the patient's desires, resulting in an individual who is happy with his or her appearance and perhaps even more motivated to practice good oral hygiene on a daily basis. With this in mind, fast-tracking the definitive treatment plan can be a critical step in overall success and patient satisfaction.

Full-mouth disinfection (FMD) represents an option to accelerate the periodontal portion of the treatment by weeks and even months, depending on the degree and severity of infection. Full-mouth disinfection requires that complete scaling and root planing be completed within 24 hours. Research has compared this therapy with partial-mouth disinfection—the traditional quadrant therapy that generally includes four appointments, two weeks apart, for a total of six weeks required to complete therapy. While success can occur with partial-mouth strategies, by and large many clinicians report mixed success due to a number of factors, and many cases that are not completed within the prescribed period. This—combined with the question of whether or not partial-mouth disinfection allows for the immune response and healing—leads one to understand the limitations of such a protocol.

Full-mouth disinfection allows for an accelerated instrumentation process that creates an environment conducive for healing and eradication of infection, while fast-tracking your aesthetic treatment plan. The research regarding this protocol included two appointments (each approximately one hour in length) with full-mouth scaling and root planing performed within 24 hours, immediately followed by oral disinfection procedures. These procedures included application of chlorhexidine to supra- and subgingival environments along with tongue brushing and mouth rinsing with chlorhexidine. Prior to this, instrumentation pockets were irrigated with a 1 percent chlorhexidine gel; after instrumentation, the following additional disinfection procedures were performed:

- Tongue-brushing for 60 seconds with a 1 percent chlorhexidine gel
- Rinsing twice with a 0.2 percent chlorhexidine solution for one minute
- Spraying the pharynx with 0.2 percent chlorhexidine
- Subgingival irrigation of all pockets three times within 10 minutes with a 1 percent chlorhexidine gel.

Subgingival application of 1 percent chlorhexidine gel was repeated at day eight. In addition to daily interdental plaque control, toothbrushing, and brushing of the dorsum of the tongue by both groups (Fig.4–1), the test populations also rinsed with and sprayed tonsils twice a day with 0.2 percent chlorhexidine for two months.

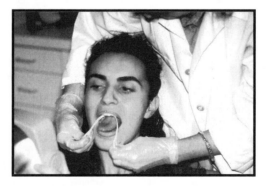

Fig. 4-1: *Brushing and dorsum of the tongue. (Courtesy of Discus Dental)*

Patients undergoing FMD exhibited both primary and secondary clinical outcomes. Primary clinical-outcome variables included an increase in clinical attachment (or alveolar bone), while secondary clinical-outcome variables included reduction in probing depths and less bleeding on probing, less inflammation, and a decrease in microbial counts. The FMD population even showed a significant reduction in probing depths and gain in clinical attachment over those receiving standard therapy.

With respect to primary clinical outcomes, the test group experienced a more significant gain in clinical attachment over the control population. These results were maintained for eight months, and in the test population, the reduction of probing depths, bleeding on probing, and gain in clinical attachment continued to improve from the baseline data. In addition, the FMD population experienced a greater reduction in spirochetes and motile bacteria, eradication of p. gingivalis, and decreased oral malodor.

Interestingly, the same research protocol was initiated without the disinfection process with chlorhexidine. The results were the same for all parameters with the exception of reduction in oral malodor. The use of chlorhexidine in varying concentrations and viscosities does not improve probing depth reduction, gain in clinical attachment, or reduction in microbial counts. The reason hypothesized for the reduction in oral malodor is that chlorhexidine neutralizes volatile sulfur compounds (VSC), the odor-producing byproduct of gram-negative bacteria, thereby eradicating bad breath. VSCs have been associated with increasing permeability of mucosa, which results in increased bacteria invasion. Most importantly, VSCs have been shown to interfere with collagen and protein synthesis. As a result, it is important to consider VSC-neutralizing agents such as chlorhexidine, zinc-containing compounds, or chlorine dioxide agents for malodor control and neutralization of harmful VSCs.

These data represent an opportunity to expand upon the original research and modify the protocol utilizing other adjunctive therapies and instrumentation techniques. For example, use of automated scalers with medicament dispensers containing a VSC-neutralizing agent could be used in place of, or in addition to, traditional hand instrumentation. Adjunctive therapies might also include the use of sub-antimicrobial doxycycline or local delivery of antimicrobial/antibiotic agents. Regardless, accelerated full-mouth debridement can be directly attributed to improved outcomes over traditional partial-mouth disinfection.

The American Dental Hygienists Association defines "optimal oral health" as a standard of health of the oral and the related tissues, which enable an individual to eat, speak, or socialize without active disease, discomfort, or embarrassment, and that contributes to general well-being and overall health. Appealing to the patient's needs—including time, tangible results and aesthetic improvements will go a long way toward achieving optimal oral health. Progressive clinicians are now in a position to offer patients a means to maximize their time and investment via FMD and other non-surgical interventions, while offering an opportunity to fast-track the aesthetic treatment plan. The result is a patient-centered approach with potential positive impact on total health.

Lasers in Dental Hygiene

by Mary Martineau, R.D.H.

Twenty-first century dental hygienists and periodontal therapists have a remarkable, cutting-edge instrument available to them that substantially enhances the treatment of periodontal disease: the diode soft tissue laser.

With the recent establishment of a distinct correlation between oral pathogenic bacteria and many serious systemic diseases, oral health has become paramount to general health. This laser is an important addition to the dental hygiene practice due to its well-documented ability to kill bacteria and debride infected tissue.

We have all heard about—and many of us have experienced—the numerous types of medical laser treatments currently available. Laser skin resurfacing, laser eye surgery, laser hair removal, and countless other laser treatments and therapies have become routine. And although the use of lasers in hygiene is gaining in popularity, it is still new and somewhat unknown to many hygienists.

Just what is a laser and how does it interact with tissue? Which laser is appropriate for use in periodontal therapy? How does the laser enhance the existing treatment of periodontal disease, and how would one incorporate a laser into their present daily hygiene practice? Those are some of the pertinent questions regarding lasers in dental hygiene. The following is a short version of an answer to those questions.

So, what is a laser, and how does it interact with tissue?

The word laser is actually an acronym for light amplification by the stimulated emission of radiation. Laser energy is essentially amplified light, and light waves emitted by lasers are a specific form of electromagnetic energy. All light is placed on the electromagnetic spectrum—the entire collection of wave energy, ranging from gamma rays to radio waves. Lasers used in dentistry sit in the infrared, non-ionizing, thermal range of the spectrum, and therefore do not cause any damage to DNA. (Fig 4–2 a, b)

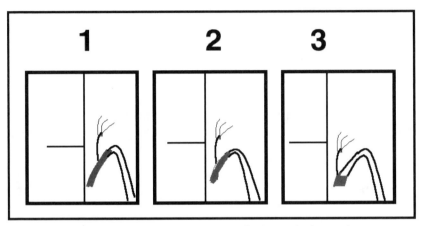

Fig. 4-2a: *Laser techniques. (Courtesy of Biolase Technology, Inc.)*

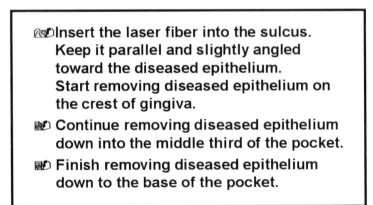

Fig. 4-2b: *Laser techniques. (Courtesy of Biolase Technology, Inc.)*

Which laser is appropriate for periodontal therapy?

Lasers are named for the rare-earth element (otherwise known as the active medium) inside them. This active medium produces a particular laser's specific interaction with a specific tissue. For example, the erbium YAG laser uses yttrium, aluminum, and garnet, doped with erbium as an active medium. Use of those elements causes the erbium YAG's energy to be highly absorbed by hydroxyapatite and water, making it an obvious choice for hard tissue cavity preparation.

Currently, the two most prevalent soft-tissue lasers in use today are the ND: YAG and the diode laser. The ND: YAG laser uses yttrium, aluminum, and garnet, doped with neodymium for its active medium. The ND: YAG laser generates a specific amplified light that is well absorbed by pigmented tissue, with some affinity for water and hemoglobin. The ND: YAG does have, however, a slight attraction to dentin as well.

The diode laser's tissue absorption characteristics are very similar to the ND: YAG, with an important distinction—no affinity to dentin. This distinction makes the diode extremely well suited for periodontal therapy work alongside the root surface of the tooth. (Fig. 4–3, a, b)

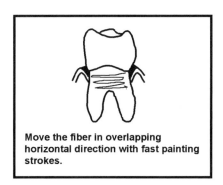

Fig. 4-3a: *Laser diodes are extremely well-suited for periodontal therapy along root surfaces.*
(Courtesy of Biolase Technology, Inc.)

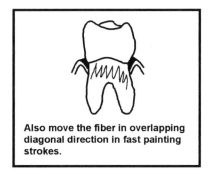

Fig. 4-3b: *Laser diodes are extremely well-suited for periodontal therapy along root surfaces.*
(Courtesy of Biolase Technology, Inc.)

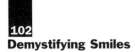

How does the diode laser enhance the treatment of periodontal disease?

Current diode lasers have FDA clearance to perform the procedure known as sulcular debridement (sometimes known as soft tissue curettage): the removal of the diseased, infected epithelial lining in the periodontal pocket. Since the most threatening oral bacteria are known to be tissue-invasive, removing them along with the infected, necrotic tissue and then cleaning the teeth have been thought to be the most effective treatment for periodontal disease. Although a professionally recognized and well-intentioned procedure, sulcular debridement, when performed with a hand curette, is not very efficient and is currently not an active part of periodontal therapy. The soft-tissue laser has emerged as the appropriate instrument to perform sulcular debridement conservatively and very effectively.

The diode laser energy has a photo-thermal action on tissue—that is to say, the light is converted into heat. This very selective and precise heat, when applied to the diseased epithelium in the sulcus, produces coagulation and then literal vaporization of the infected tissue. Some research indicates that a biostimulation effect occurs in the underlying tissue, which seems to stimulate healing. Also, since anaerobic pathogens have a dark pigmentation, the laser energy vaporizes them as well. Of course, there are variables to consider when using a laser—for instance, how high the power is set, whether the beam is pulsed or continuous, and how long the beam is allowed to be in contact with the tissue.

How would one incorporate a laser into their present daily hygiene practice?

It is important to know how laser energy works in order to use it effectively. In fact, formal training and certification are required for anyone to legally use a laser on patients, and this book is by no means a substitute for this or any other required education. The training includes more detailed science and some basic physics of laser energy as well as hands-on laser work. At the time of this writing, not all states allowed hygienists to perform laser-assisted hygiene. Generally speaking, the states that allow a hygienist to perform sulcular debridement with a curette allow hygienists to perform that same procedure using a laser—provided, of course, they have completed the necessary training.

Laser hygiene still involves curettes and the ultrasonic scaler—they're still used to debride the teeth. The laser is then used to debride the diseased, necrotic, epithelial lining of the pocket. (Some clinicians debride the epithelial wall first and then debride the teeth.) Laser therapy takes about 10 to15 seconds per pocket surface (10 to15 seconds to debride the lingual epithelial wall of one tooth from mesial to distal; the same for the facial epithelial wall.)

Of the several diode lasers currently on the market, most are about the size of a breadbox and simply plug into the wall. The energy beam is emitted through fiber-optic tubing that is usually 400 microns in diameter and is slipped into an aluminum auto-clavable handpiece.

Since oral bleeding allows bacteria to enter the blood stream—bacteria that can permeate the tissue to potentially create a serious threat to the general health of the people that we treat—logic dictates that we remove the pathologic bacteria from the sulcus of our patient's mouths along with debriding the teeth. This is critical. The diode laser provides dental hygienists with a viable, precise, safe instrument to do just that.

Laser procedures

The goals of laser technology are to promote wound-healing, hemostatsis, reduce the number of cultivated bacteria, and melt or vaporize tissue without inducing irreversible damage to adjacent tissue. The sequence of treatment is as follows:

- Laser safety glasses for clinician and patient

- Review pocket depths

- Patient is anesthetized (optional)

- Ultrasonic instrumentation and hand instrumentation (scaling and root planing)

- Conventional bacterial decontamination and antimicrobial irrigation before and after laser therapy (have the patient rinse with an appropriate mouth rinse)

- Turn unit on; initiate the tip; hold handpiece gently

- Remove epithelial lining with the laser by measuring fiber tip to base of pocket. Use a sweeping motion away from the tooth and towards tissue pocket wall—not against the tooth surface

- Constantly move the fiber tip for 20-60 seconds to achieve laser bacterial decontamination

- Wipe debris off the tip frequently to prevent overheating

- Dispense post-operative written and oral self-care instructions

Gingival Aesthetics

Many articles and clinical features involving aesthetic dentistry include the shape, the color, the position, and/or characteristics of the teeth. Often in this discussion, the gingiva and its effect on the beauty of a smile are overlooked. Yet, there are probably at least four areas involving gingival aesthetics that can be easily evaluated during the dental hygiene pre-diagnosis session. Consideration should be given to the following:

- Standard for excellence of gingival health and the health of the surrounding structures

- Levels of gingival crests (crown lengthening)

- Excessive gingival display (gummy smile)

- Gingival embrasures (black triangle)

The aesthetic result depends upon proper soft-tissue management. The fundamental principles of aesthetics must be cemented in a disease-free oral cavity with a strong emphasis in prevention, attention to the patient's total health, and facilitation of the patient's desires and the practice's services.

A dental hygienist cannot pay lip service to a standard of excellence for the periodontal tissue and surrounding structures—the tissue must be *ideal*. Ideal gingival health is 0-3 mm pockets and no bleeding upon provocation; in other words, an oral stage that has *zilch* in terms of disease. There must be full assessment, 6-point periodontal charting and/or graphing, care planning, treatment, and evaluation completed on every patient under a "no excuse" clause. This means that every dental hygienist, with the support of their dental practice, must commit the time and energy needed to establish and maintain a disease-free environment. It is our responsibility to report to the restorative dentist and patient our pre-diagnosis periodontal summary and treatment plan. Hygiene services must not stop—whether they are provided in your practice or referred to an oral health partner—nor must any aesthetic modalities begin until ideal tissue results are achieved.

In addition, paying attention to the gingival margin lines can make a world of difference to the outcome of aesthetic treatments. The gingival levels should radiate symmetry and balance. Symmetry should be established at the gingival margins of each contralateral tooth from the central to the second molars. The gingival crest of the lateral incisors should be approximately 1mm below the crest of the central incisors, and the crest of the canines should be equal to that of the central incisors. The remaining posterior teeth should follow a natural graduation in appearance from canine to second molar. (See Fig. 3-2, Chapter 2)

A scenario that relates to the height of the gingival crests is when a patient says, "Some of my teeth are shorter than the others." After your examination, you measure with a ruler and discover that teeth #8, 7, and 6 have a reduced crown length due to excessive gingival coverage. What your patient is saying is that she is dissatisfied with her visual perception of the difference in lengths of their clinical crowns. This discrepancy is generally better corrected prior to the beginning of restorative therapy. In some cases, however, after minor gingival recontouring has been performed (with no violation of the biological width, which I will discuss under "Gingival Embrasure"), the patient may decide that she is happy with the outcome—and that is all that is desired.

When assessing a patient for aesthetic modalities, the face, lips, and smile must all be considered. The teeth should be in the center of the mouth with no distractions. The upper lip should fall near the maxillary gingival line, and the lower lip should cradle the maxillary incisal plane. If the teeth are not in the middle of the smile, there may be excessive gingival display when smiling. This gingival-to-lip relationship is often termed a gummy smile. Generally, that is defined as any patient who shows more than 2 mm of gingival during a full smile. The etiologies of such a condition are beyond the scope of this section, but may include a short or hyperactive lip, an altered passive eruption, dentoalveolar extrusion, and/or vertical maxillary excess. In terms of excess gingival display, it also needs to be remedied before any definitive therapy. The anatomic crown hidden prior to the surgery (and exposed after) will affect the visual presence and the restorative-gingival margin interface.

Additionally, the appearance of the interdental papilla must also be considered when attempting to achieve optimal effects. The papilla must fill in the interproximal spaces. Open gingival embrasures (black triangles) may occur for a variety of reasons—the shape of the crown (contour and contact point), root angulations (the roots are not parallel or straight), and interproximal bone loss due to periodontal disease and or recession/iatrogenic insult. These conditions make the papilla unable to fill the entire embrasure space and cause disharmony of the smile. Correctional treatments of open gingival embrasures may involve one or any combination of orthodontic therapy, periodontal therapy, and refabrication of the restoration.

Biological width is a term used to describe the approximate 3 mm distance from the gingival crest to the crest of the alveolar bone. It is measured by "sounding the bone." After profound anesthesia has been administered, a periodontal probe is placed midfacially on a central incisor and pushed through the attachment apparatus until the alveolar crest is found. A situation of high crest occurs when less that 3 mm distance is determined from the gingival margin to the alveolar crest; a low crest distance occurs when the gingival crest to the alveolar crest is less than 3 mm. Therefore, before beginning any restorative treatment, each patient must be evaluated to establish his or her own attachment height, which is determined by subtracting the true sulcus (measured sulcus depth minus 0.5 mm for penetration of the probe) from the sounding depth (measurement from the free gingival margin to the osseous crest.)

In restorative options, the location of the margin relative to the bone and height of the attachment is crucial. If this is not considered, and the restoration violates the biological width, you have a dental hygienist's nightmare! Biological width invasion results in poor gingival health, which breaches the standard of excellence for gingival tissues. It also remains unresolved until the defective restoration is replaced.

Simply stated: Aesthetic balance and symmetry cannot be accomplished in a mouth if the teeth or tissue are in the wrong place. A comprehensive treatment plan that includes techniques for the preservation or correction of gingival architecture involves interdisciplinary care. The dental hygiene analysis of the patient's smile incorporates all aspects of the dentition. The soft tissue must be assessed for health, contour, and measure of display in order to facilitate a pleasing smile for our patients.

Strategies for Non-Surgical Therapy Program

Calibration. Minimize the ported 1 mm-3 mm margin for error between practitioners by setting up quarterly calibration meetings. Ensure that all dental hygienists and doctors exert the same amount of pressure during full-mouth probing (15-20 gms is optimal).

Make sure the periodontal treatment plan is not considered the ugly stepsister to complete dentistry. One option is to include it in the total restorative treatment fee—perhaps even including one year (four sessions) at no cost once definitive restorations are seated. For example, if your practice charges $2,400 to $4,000 to provide non-surgical periodontal therapy and post-hygiene renewal and management sessions, have the fee include anything the hygienist needs to do or use to treat the patient, including laser therapy, irrigation, polishing agents, and all appropriate self-service products to support the oral health.

Words we use. Root planing and scaling paint no picture in patients' minds as to the outcome of the service. Terms like debridement and detoxify illustrate results.

Are all new patients seen first by the dentist? Think through the patients who have not been seen in the office for a long period of time (two to three years). Where should they be scheduled when they call the office? Will they qualify for a new-patient examination prior to a hygiene session? If the patient lands in the hygiene schedule, does the dental hygienist have the knowledge and ability to take a step back (without fear of negative ramifications) to perform cursory pre-diagnostics services? What protocols are in place if the hygienist determines that the patient needs more than "just a cleaning?"

Practices need to think about hygiene in the same terms as restorative care. If a patient entered the office with a broken tooth and, after examination, it was determined that he or she needed endodontics, post and core, a crown, and crown lengthening, would the treating doctor proceed without discussing the treatment sequence first—and without discussing fees? Probably not. Why is it expected, then, that a hygienist will just clean up an overdue patient, or constantly work in a bloody environment, while attempting to perform non-surgical therapy? Why should he or she charge for a just a cleaning (while permitted an inadequate amount of time to perform the therapy), only to have the examining dentist come in and say, "Everything looks great—see you in six months?" Who makes the differential diagnosis—and schedules accordingly—when patients call? Is it left to the judgment of the treatment coordinator?

Establish schedule templates and treatment protocols and allow for overdue patients (especially after reviewing hygiene notes while the patient is engaged in conversation on the telephone). If the patient is scheduled for more time then clinically needed to perform the therapeutic service, the remaining time can always be spent on educating and enrolling him or her in advances in dentistry and oral health. Or when was the last time a patient enjoyed a shorter amount of time in the clinical chair? What an unexpected pleasure to be able to leave—not on time—but earlier than planned!

Stay tuned to future ultrasonic trends. Expanded applications of ultrasonics will use low power, small inserts with innovative techniques and chemotherapeutic agents. To learn how we use ultrasonics, and why its rapidly changing, enroll in a reputable lecture and hands-on program to discover all the newest trends in delivery of care that promote periodontal healing and safeguard restorative dentistry.

Consultation appointments. Why is it that when a patient needs restorative dentistry, he or she is rescheduled for a consultation appointment? But if that patient "only" needs periodontal therapy, then the financial arrangements and sessions are scheduled at the front desk—without a consultation. Shouldn't periodontal health be on par with restorative needs and require an additional consultation appointment? Since periodontal disease is *not* treatable—just manageable—why not stress the importance of a disease-free oral environment at all times?

Do not close your mind and believe that the field of aesthetics is of no use to you if you work in a specialty practice—a periodontal practice, for instance.

If your office shares patients with an aesthetic-specialty practice for periodontal management appointments—or, the reverse, if you work in an aesthetic practice and refer to a periodontal office—you need to make sure that patients have care plans coordinated with their interdisciplinary network of offices. This guarantees that preventive management protocols complement each other: The patient receives the same self-care message from *all* locations, and no one is unintentionally damaging or neglecting the needs of the restorative work.

How many times does a hygienist perform a #01110 on patients when they actually have bleeding and even suppuration? If a prophy is an appointment meant to manage health and the patient is not healthy—well, then what are we really maintaining?

"Why was it always a 'cleaning,' and now I need non-surgical periodontal therapy?" What rationales should a clinician include in the patient response?

- Strong, emerging research and a connection between oral health and systemic health, such as low birth weights, pre-term delivery, diabetes, heart disease, etc.

- Reduces or detoxifies the oral cavity

- Minimizes or eliminate hemorrhaging

- Improves immune response to fighting off other systemic infections

- Treatment and management of incurable diseases/infections

- Aids in the prevention of future setback or outbreaks of active disease

- Possibility of bone repair

- Improves bad breath and overall appearance of the teeth and gums

> **Periodontal and Occlusal Strategy:**
>
> *If a tooth, sextant, or quadrant shows characteristics of localized periodontal infection (loss of attachment and reduced alveolar support),take a closer look at the occlusal forces. The diseased area may also be experiencing secondary occlusal trauma. Clinical signs may include tooth mobility, migration, excessive spacing, compromised function, and gingival recession. (Refer to Chapter 1, "Merging of the Occlusion"*

Sequencing of treatment (no more drive-by dentistry)

1. Periodontal therapy and health or stabilization
2. Fabrication of provisional therapies
3. Maturation of the biologic width followed by final margin placement
4. Case re-evaluation
5. Construction of final case
6. Excellent laboratory communication

The Association of Dental Implant Auxiliaries and Practice Management and Dental Hygiene

By Ann-Marie C. DePalma, R.D.H., B.S.

For those who practice implant dentistry, the International Congress of Oral Implantologists (ICOI) has, for the last 30 years, provided extensive information about this craft. As the largest implant organization worldwide, ICOC has enhanced the educational base of implantologists.

It is also the only implant association that has a component association for dental auxiliaries, hygienists, assistants, and front office staff. The mission of the Association of Dental Implant Auxiliaries and Practice Management (ADIA and PM) is to develop educational criteria and programs to expand auxiliaries' contributions to the field of implant dentistry.

The ADIA consists of a network of team members who share the common goal of high-quality continuing education at both local and national levels. In addition to continuing education programs, ADIA provides informational resources and special recognition for implant training, as well as access to ADIA and ICOI newsletters and journals.

One of the ADIA continuing education programs is the Dental Hygiene Implant Certification Program (DHICP). This comprehensive program provides an overview of implantology, designed for all team members. It covers surgical, prosthetic, and maintenance considerations, reviews treatment planning for implant patients, and provides the entire team with the verbal and interdisciplinary skills needed to work effectively with implant patients. You could call it the basic nuts and bolts of implants!

Also available through ADIA is the office and business management program, designed to educate participants regarding the non-clinical aspects of dental implantology. Topics covered in this program give all auxiliaries an overview of practice management as it relates to implants. Areas covered include case presentations and frequently-asked questions, financial arrangements, the use of dental and medical insurance, patient motivation, and marketing. Both the DHICP and the business management program are designed to give the staff the knowledge they need to enhance all aspects of the dental implant practice.

Another aspect of ADIA is its credentialing program. Membership in ADIA and PM is open to any office management or clinical dental team member; each member may then undertake advanced levels of certification. These higher recognition levels reward commitment on the part of the auxiliary who wants to be more actively involved in the implant dentistry. Advanced membership levels include certified member, advanced certified member, and fellowship status. To gain each level, the dental team member must meet certain criteria. These include attending DHICP programs, committing to other dental continuing educational programs offered by various sponsors (of which a certain percentage is directly related to implants), and demonstration of activities within organized implant dentistry. These credentialing levels allow participants to demonstrate to the rest of the dental profession achievement and commitment to the field of oral implantology.

For dental hygienists, continuing education is an ongoing part of our clinical practice. Depending on your state's rules and regulations, continuing educational programs are required to advance education and maintain the health of the patients we see. The ADIA provides a unique opportunity for the hygienist to gain valuable knowledge regarding implant dentistry, a field that is constantly evolving.

The following information from the ADIA can be used as in-office material for dental implant patients.

Evaluating Implants for Success and Failure

by Lynn D. Mortilla, R.D.H.
Reprinted from Implants News & Views, *Vol.2, No. 3, for the* ADIA & PM Newsletter

Judging the success or failure of implants involves more than just evaluating whether the implant is retained (and restored) or removed. Many clinicians have determined ways to evaluate the success of dental implants, and there are many factors defining the parameters to judge implant success.

An important point to remember is that implants are not teeth, and so many traditional methods utilized to judge the health and success of teeth vary and differ for diagnosing and treating dental implants. The American Dental Association Council on Dental Materials, Instruments, and Equipment evaluates the effect that implants have on adjacent teeth, function, aesthetics, presence of infection, discomfort, paresthesia, intrusion of mandibular canal, and patient satisfaction. Dr. Carl Misch, pioneer in implant dentistry, cites the following criteria to gauge implant success.

Longevity. Dr. Misch's clinical criteria for success are 90 percent for five years and 85 percent for 10 years. Statistics should include all implants placed. Tallies should be drawn from the day the implants were inserted—not post-prosthetic placement.

Pain. Temperature changes are often indicative of a problem with teeth. Such early warning signs are not present with dental implants. With healthy dental implants, there is usually an absence of pain under horizontal and vertical stress. Presence of pain could indicate nerve impingement or mobility. If a patient experiences sensitivity, an evaluation of load and function is necessary. Occlusion and parafunctional habits may be to blame. There may be a need to add more implants or modify the prosthesis to correct the problem and eliminate the source of pain. Aggressive occlusal adjustments and/or occlusal splint therapy may be indicated. If the patient still experiences pain, the prognosis is usually poor and the patient should be questioned as to the severity of pain. If the pain is significant, the implant should be removed.

Rigid fixation. Mobile implants should not be restored. Often, mobility of a prosthesis or a prosthetic component can mimic implant mobility. Osteointegration is the direct contact of bone to implant at the light microscope level. There is no specified percentage of bone that needs to be in contact with the implant to assure success. Unlike the situation with teeth, mobility is a primary consideration in determining implant health and longevity. Since implants do not have a periodontal ligament, and consequently act like an ankylosed tooth, absence of clinical mobility under load is an important criterion for success.

Percussion. Percussion gives no indication of health or disease around an implant, but can help diagnose sensitivity.

Bone loss. Properly evaluating crestal bone has become a hallmark of implant success, but evaluating bone depth with probing levels and radiographs poses a challenge to many clinicians.

The distance between implant threads is generally 0.6mm. This is a good radiographic marker since bone around implants is usually gauged in 0.5 mm increments. However, bone loss must be taken into account. Early bone loss is usually the result of excessive stress. Also, immature bone near the crest can be lost due to improper occlusion or parafunctional habits. Occlusal modifications and splints may be utilized. After an abutment is attached to an implant, 0.5 mm of connective tissue will form apical to the abutment-implant junction. Generally, there is bone loss to the first thread of the implant within the first year of function. Yearly clinical assessments of bone loss in increments greater than 0.5 mm need to be diagnosed, documented, and sometimes treated. When half an implant's height has bone loss, it is considered a failure.

Radiographic evaluation. It is often a challenge to expose a good clinical x-ray of an implant. Often, the implant apex surpasses the apex of teeth. Film placement is hindered by muscle attachments and intraoral anatomy and can lead to foreshortened periapicals, which serve no diagnostic value.

To monitor crestal bone, vertical bitewings are the best choice. If a periapical is exposed, the apical region may be omitted to check crestal bone levels. If the x-ray shows clear threads, the angulation was accurate. Any sign of blurry threads are not diagnostically acceptable to monitor crestal bone loss. A radiolucency circumferential to the implant is indicative of soft-tissue encapsulation due to infection, iatrogenic procedures, mobility, or poor bone healing. The prognosis for these situations is poor. A radiolucency at the implant apex could be indicative of an alveolar perforation, use of a contaminated drill, overheating of the bone, or infection. These may be able to be treated with surgical correction.

Baseline radiographs should be taken the day of prosthesis delivery; six-months post-prosthesis delivery, and one-year post-delivery. If there are no radiographic changes, an x-ray should be taken every three years. If there are signs of pathology, clinical symptoms, mobility problems, or advanced bone loss, diagnosis and treatment should be initiated and an x-ray should be taken every six months for one year after the problem has ceased or been corrected.

Peri-implant disease. Peri-implantitis is bone loss around an implant. Its common etiology is stress or bacteria. If bone loss is created by stress, there will be no bacteria present, but the pocket created can provide a perfect home for anaerobic bacteria, which can be responsible for continued bone loss even if the stress is removed.

The lack of a connective tissue barrier around implants creates a unique situation. A lack of these fibers means bacteria have an easier path of entry to destroy bone. The presence of exudate indicates some type of infection. Treatment with short-term systemic antibiotics and topical chlorhexadine is the best initial approach. If the exudate is present for more than two weeks or frequently reoccurs, a surgical correction may be necessary.

Probing depth. Probing around implants is a controversial topic. The standard safe pressure at which to probe is 20 grams. Plastic, pressure-sensitive probes are the best tools to determine implant sulcus depth. A fixed reference point should be utilized to eliminate inaccurate probing depths due to gingival hyperplasia and hypertrophy. Dentate patients generally have deeper probing depths than edentulous patients. Since there is no connective tissue attachment zone around implants, the probe is in much closer contact to the bone. It is important to avoid introducing bacteria (seeding) into the sulcus around implants. Dipping the probe in chlorhexadine before use in an implant sulcus site is advantageous.

As with teeth, pockets greater than 4 mm are very difficult for a patient to maintain, but it is often difficult to obtain accurate probing depths due to prosthesis design. Probing should be performed in the presence of bone loss (for monitoring purposes) or pathology. Probing can also give valuable information regarding tissue consistency, bleeding, and/or exudate. Since x-rays can only judge mesial-distal bone levels, probing can aid in assessing facial-lingual bone levels.

Bleeding index. There are fewer blood vessels around implants than around teeth. By itself, bleeding is not the most reliable indicator, since impingement on well-adapted permucosal tissue and excessive probing pressure can precipitate false-positive results. The presence of plaque and/or ulcerated sulcular epithelium is the better indicator of a problem.

In any and all cases, evaluating and assessing the presence or lack of health are the first steps to treating implant complications. Success comes from the interaction of many variables, including concordance with the patient. Surgical technique, good prosthetics, good oral hygiene, and timely maintenance appointments enhance the success of dental implants. Documentation is imperative to monitor progress and identify potential problems.

Association of Dental Implant Auxiliaries and Practice Management Auxiliaries' Aide Dental Implant Assessment and Oral Hygiene Recommendations

Name:

Date:

X-Rays:
Dental Implants:
  Area(s) UR UA UL LR LA LL
  Quantity
  Type of Implant
  Type of Prosthesis
  Types of Implant: Types of Prosthesis:

RF = Root Form CCB = Cement Retained Crown/Bridge
B = Blade SCB = Screw Retained Crown/Bridge
S = Subperiosteal OD = Overdenture

Calculus: Supragingival Negligible Light Moderate Heavy
Subgingival: Negligible Light Moderate Heavy
Plaque: Negligible Light Moderate Heavy
Debris: Negligible Light Moderate Heavy
Gingival Condition/Color: Pink Red Cyanotic
Edema: Slight Extensive Interdental Generalized
Consistency:: Firm Spongy Hyperplastic Friable
Papillae: Blunted Cratered Enlarged
Bleeding: Slight Moderate Heavy
Exudate Areas:
Recession Areas:
Comments:

Mobility:
Occlusion:

Fig. 4–4: *ADIA and PM assessment and oral hygiene recommendations form.*

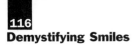

Association of Dental Implant Auxiliaries and
Practice Management
Dental Implant Assessment and Oral Hygiene Recommendations
Auxiliaries' Aide
Oral Hygiene Instruction/Aids

Manual Toothbrush:
Automatic Toothbrush:
Specialty Toothbrush:
Floss:
Intra-dental Device:
Oral Irrigator:
Dentifrice:
Chemotherapeutic Mouthrinse:
Areas of Concern:

Recare Interval Recommended:_____months ———— * ————

As part of your dental treatment, you will receive/have received dental implants. The long-term health and success of your dental implants depend largely on your ability to keep them free of bacterial plaque. Following the routine hygiene schedule we have given you is also extremely important so we can monitor and evaluate your oral health and professionally care for your teeth and implants. We will make recommendations to you relating to the products and personal at-home hygiene program that will suit your dental needs.

Fig. 4–5: *ADIA and PM oral hygiene and instruction aids.*

Association of Dental Implant Auxiliaries and Practice Management
Auxiliaries' Aide
Dental Implant Evaluation & Assessment Report

Patient: Date:
Recare Interval: Last Recare
Appointment:
Medical History Update:
Oral Hygiene Assessment:
Hard and Soft Tissue Evaluation Clinical and Radiographic
Findings:
Prosthetic Concerns:
X Rays Enclosed:

_____I have suggested the patient make an appointment
to see you for implant evaluation.

_____Please provide us with a copy of your most current
panoramic radiograph of this patient.
Sincerely,

Fig. 4–6: *ADIA and PM dental implant evaluation and assessment report.*

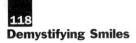

Making a Difference in My Little Corner of the World

by Karen Stueve, R.D.H.

I graduated from dental hygiene school in 1981 and came away from that experience with a sincere hatred for periodontal disease.

I didn't understand it very well back then, as I believe most of the dental world did not. One thing I did know, though, was that I wanted to make a difference in my patients' lives, and as a dental hygienist, I have always tried to live up to that goal.

While in hygiene school, I ran across an obscure reference to a belief that there was some connection between periodontal disease and heart disease. Then my father died in 1991; he had heart disease, and at that point, had survived two heart attacks. He also had periodontal disease, which, unfortunately, was never resolved before his death from congestive heart failure. But from that time, I kept a file of articles with any mention of a connection between periodontal disease and any other systemic disease.

At a staff meeting one day, we were discussing how to market the practice to attract new patients. All the usual suspects were rounded up—go to the schools and talk with kids, run ads in the yellow pages, ask patients for referrals, etc. While all these things are fine, I wanted to do something really different and, I hoped, meaningful. My idea was to put together a packet of information about the connection between periodontal disease and systemic diseases, along with information about our office and our excellent periodontal therapy program, including a referral pad, much like the ones we use to refer our patients to specialists. We would hand-deliver or send these packets to local physicians, cardiologists, and OB/GYNs, hoping to garner referrals, or at least to encourage them to recommend that their patients see their dentists and ask to have examinations for periodontal disease.

The outcome of that meeting was what I call the Physician Referral Packet. It consists of a red, two-pocket folder with a label on the front that proclaims: THE CONNECTION: The link between periodontal disease and other systemic diseases.

The practice's business card goes inside one front pocket. Inside the left front pocket is an introductory letter explaining the periodontal program in our practice, the purpose of the packet, and a request that the physicians please encourage their patients to ask for exams for gum disease. I also enclosed a copy of our protocol to treat Case Type 3 periodontal patients. This pocket also contained a pad with referral slips to our office. On the right side are several pamphlets, a study about the connection of periodontal disease and cardiovascular disease, and a wonderful article written by Shirley Gutkowski, R.D.H., B.S. on the assessment of periodontal disease in a healthcare environment.

After *RDH* magazine published an article about this project, Shirley Gutkowski and I received requests for information on the packet from all over the country. I am keeping in touch with these people via e-mail and by updating two e-mail groups that I belong to as we get response to the packet from local physicians.

June 18, 2001

Dear Dr. _____:

I recently saw your patient [name] for a new patient examination, comprehensive exam for periodontal disease, oral cancer screening, and full mouth x-rays. [Name] made this appointment after your recommendation that he see a dentist. I have enclosed a copy of his periodontal chart showing the diseased areas as brown lines, red ovals as bleeding areas, and blue lines as healthy areas. Four decayed teeth were found and restored, and I have recommended removal of the wisdom teeth after the gum disease is under control.

[Name's] periodontal examination reveals that he has moderate periodontal disease with 4, 5, and 6-millimeter pockets and severe inflammation of the gingival. I have recommended a series of periodontal therapy appointments followed by a prescription of doxycycline to remove the offending bacteria from the gums and throughout the body. He will be taught how to maintain the health of his gums for a lifetime so that these harmful bacteria will no longer find their way into the bloodstream.

As you are probably aware, periodontal disease is usually painless, and many times there are no significant outward symptoms. This makes it important for everyone to have a comprehensive examination for periodontal disease by a dentist to determine if disease is present.

I appreciate your referral of [name] to a dentist. In light of recent research connecting periodontal disease with heart disease, diabetes, and other systemic diseases, it is important that we, as healthcare providers, work together to give our patients every advantage in returning to health.

Sincerely,
Jeffery R. VanTreese, D.D.S.

Enclosure

Fig. 4–7: *Example letter, sent pretreatment.*

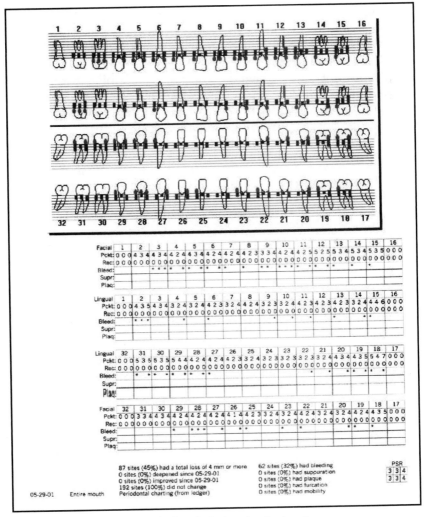

Fig. 4–8: *Sample chart, sent pretreatment.*

June 30, 2001

Dear Dr. _____

My name is Karen Stueve, and I am a dental hygienist in the employ of Dr. Jeff VanTreese. I have been treating our mutual patient, [name], for his periodontal disease. Recently, he completed a series of non-surgical periodontal therapy appointments, and I have enclosed a copy of his most recent periodontal charting, and some before and after photos of his gums. As you can see, his gums have healed very nicely; he has fewer pockets and much less bleeding on probing.

He will now be seen every three months and will be carefully monitored to be sure that his periodontal condition has been stabilized. If he follows our home-care instructions and stays on a regular periodontal maintenance schedule, he should be able to maintain the health of his gums for a lifetime.

Thank you so much for referring [name]. It is always a pleasure to help someone achieve better health and eliminate one of the risk factors for heart disease. With new research verifying the connection between periodontal disease and systemic diseases, it is important for everyone to have regular examinations for periodontal disease. Most people show no visible signs of gum disease, and we would welcome the opportunity to assist your patients in achieving optimal health.

Yours in better health,

Karen L. Stueve, R.D.H.

Enclosure

Fig. 4–9: *Example letter, sent post-treatment.*

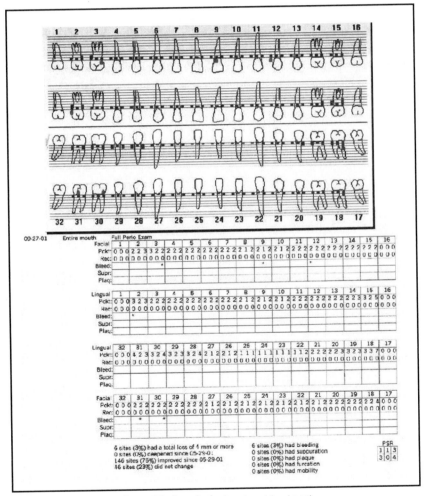

Fig. 4–10: *Sample chart sent post-treatment.*

Create Your Strategies

Change is happening faster than ever before, and we can't afford to let it just happen. • **Marsha Farnsworth Richie**

    This exercise, provided at the end of each chapter, is to assist you in designing a game plan in order to develop the skills, knowledge, and expertise necessary to propel you to your next level of personal and professional growth. Ask, answer, and record:

My periodontal-balance goals for the future are:

_____

_____

_____

The areas for which I would like assistance and support to achieve my goals are:

_____

_____

_____

My action steps to get in the game and achieve those goals are:

_____

_____

_____

My list of specific goals and the dates I wish to accomplish them includes:

_____

_____

_____

Possible obstacles to watch out for (*i.e.,* fear of rejection, fear of change, and lack of accountability, denial, lack of focus, lack of self-evaluation, lack of mentoring relationships):

_____

_____

_____

FIVE

Clinical Delivery: Smile Preserving Programs

If you see a bandwagon, it's too late. • **Sir James Goldsmith**

Hygiene Debriefing

One of the clinical changes we must undertake is to commit to comprehensive patient assessment before performing diagnosis and treatment.

- *Smile design:* Establish a basis for restorative and aesthetic treatment planning, such as aesthetic concerns, and oral-health goals.

- *Functional considerations:* Gather information and clinically note signs and symptoms that could affect preventive and restorative care—occlusal discrepancies, muscles of mastication, and temporal-mandibular joints.

- *Hygiene clinical delivery:* Track recare schedules and appropriate armamentarium and modalities.

- *Restorative possibilities:* Communicate areas of concern, treatment options, benefits, and risks.

- *Self-care products:* Record information on self-care habits—how, when, how much, etc.

When designing a hygiene-care plan, have an expanded frame of reference—including full-mouth restoration and aesthetic services—to provide new dimensions for the dental hygienist. Like a complicated organism, the dental hygiene-care plan and the comprehensive restorative-treatment plan integrate different valuable pieces. However, they only have power when linked together. The totality of interrelated phases makes the hygiene and dental methods of care succeed. Since aesthetics is changing our professions, it must be included, so the complexities of the interconnected programs are further challenged.

The hygiene-aesthetic care plan, a component of the complete hygiene-care plan, is a written proposal that directs the dental hygienist and the patient as they work together to meet or exceed the patient's goals for aesthetics. Predominantly, the plan individualizes care, keeps focus on the patient's long-term outcomes for oral health and smile, establishes interventions and a sequence of care, and monitors the patient's progress. This is all facilitated while ensuring continuity of care and communication among the oral heath professionals involved. Interventions, such as patient education, oral disease prevention, oral health behaviors, health promotion strategies, and professional armamentarium, are formulated into the plan.

Professional armamentarium

Since improper professional and patient self-care can adversely affect the longevity and appearance of cosmetic and aesthetic restorations, some basic principles should be adhered to in order to preserve the substance and beauty of the service. For instance, while a majority of hygienists have a level of proficiency in instrument sharpening, few have mastered the clinical angulations or embraced the importance of a sharp curette. Automatic instrument-sharpening machines are worth learning about and investing in. They provide the clinician with easy sharpening so that a multitude of clinicians can sharpen the same instrument with equal results. (If you were like me in school, you never quite understood hand-sharpening instruments via shadows and a sun dial!)

Dull curettes may ditch and/or scratch the surface of a tooth-colored restoration, and the majority of information concerning hand instrumentation of tooth-colored restorations concludes that sharp curettes offer the tactile sensitivity necessary to debride without scratching the aesthetic materials. In addition, a gentle, horizontal stroke rather than a heavy up-and-down stroke should be applied to safeguard the integrity of a bonded margin. Some of the newer plastic instruments (with streamlined shanks and blades) may also be considered for debriding. These can be sharpened with material-specific sharpening stones. These new additions provide a welcome advantage over the original plastic designs that needed to be thrown out after a few uses and sterilization processes.

Another instrument consideration is, "How sharp is your explorer?" Or, a better question would be, "How *old* is your explorer?" If you are using an explorer during your aesthetic, caries, and/or periodontal assessments, it needs to be replaced on a regular basis, because it will not retain sharpness and diagnostic/tactile properties. Restorative margins should be treated with care, and running a dull explorer over the restoration edges is not the most favorable approach to determining its location.

Being Careful or Being Real?

Posted on a dental hygienist e-mail network was a scenario that went something like this:

"I received a notation from our periodontal-prostheticentist not to use ultrasonic (microsonics) near the margins of crowns he had done on a patient, since it might damage or change them." The hygienist who posted this e-mail was looking for confirmation as to whether or not the dentist was being "too careful" or "unreal."

I admit that, at times, I spend too much time on the internet, but please—be careful whose advice from the computer you take!

This question poses a perfect opportunity to plan professional strategy by picking up the phone and calling the referring doctor. Schedule a time to discuss care of restorative dentistry. Open up the channels of communication.

In the arena of high-tech instrumentation, it is suggested that ultrasonic and sonic scalers and air abrasion units not be used on or around a tooth with a tooth-colored restoration. Ultrasonic and sonic scalers should be avoided on the margins of any restorations—tooth-colored or amalgam; apical or coronal to the margin may be acceptable if the clinician is proficiently trained in effective ultrasonic debridement techniques. Air-abrasive techniques can scratch and pit the surface of a restoration, therefore making it more susceptible to plaque accumulation and staining.

Research in the areas of hygiene instrumentation and aesthetic treatment is encouraging; however, long-term clinical relevance needs to be further explored. The bottom line is that continual, inappropriate professional care at repeated three, four, and/or six-month recare appointments may be a powerful contributor to marginal breakdown and early "cosmetic" failure of tooth-colored treatments.

Sodium fluoride treatments delivered after aesthetic recare, and definitive restorative placement and as part of self-care habits, should be components of a smile-preserving program. Acidulated phosphate fluoride and stannous fluoride should not be used when patients have tooth-colored restorations. Acidulated phosphate fluoride has been shown to etch porcelain and may affect the filler particles in composite resins. Stannous fluoride may also cause discoloration of the restorations.

Hygiene-care plans, customized interventions, and smile-preserving sessions provide more opportunities for professional growth and best practices for a cosmetic office. It is simply no longer appropriate to negate these stages of the hygiene process of care. Just as it is inappropriate to hold on to the belief that calculus causes periodontal disease, it is now just as inappropriate to leave aesthetic treatment care only to the restorative team. What is appropriate is to make restorative dentistry and supportive aesthetic hygiene services interrelated for our patients.

Polishing

Properly polishing and maintaining restorative treatments are services that can preserve and prolong their longevity. However, selecting the right polishing systems for the total smile can be difficult. Because of the differences in the size, shape, number of filler particles, type of resin, varying porcelain/ceramic materials, and the properties of adhesion to natural tooth structures, one system may be incapable of creating a high shine on all aesthetic solutions.

Differentiating among restorative options guides a clinician to those polishing agents to use and what results to expect. This will save time, for example, in trying to reproduce a high gloss on a material that never had one. Generally, to bring a surface gloss to restorations, a polishing system includes the application of aluminum oxide or diamond paste. If you are having trouble getting the desired results with your current methods, check with the manufacturer of the restorative material for polishing guidelines and product suggestions. Studies suggest that pairing a specific restorative material with a matching polishing system produces the smoothest surface.

There is information (scanning electron magnification images, or SEMS) that shows that conventional prophy paste roughens, scratches, and dulls the surfaces of tooth-colored restorative materials and, possibly, restorative margins. Coarse prophy paste may also cause premature plucking of glass or silica filler particles from the resin matrix (organic paste) of composites, leaving a porous surface texture. This may cause excessive wear, staining, and premature breakdown of the restoration.

The literature is not consistent on the subject of polishing cups versus prophy cups. Some sources state that polishing pastes should be used on flexible buffing cups, points, or discs/wheels rather than regular prophy cups. It has been suggested that regular prophy cups may generate too much heat and cause damage to the composite materials. However, other reports suggest that latch-type, webbed prophy cups tend to polish as well as those in disposable prophy angles. Faced with rival approaches—what should the foot soldiers of aesthetic hygiene do?

I recommend using buffing cups or points when performing aesthetic polishing. If not available, the next choice would be soft-webbed prophy cups.

Begin the process by determining the extent of polishing necessary, evaluating the restoration and tooth stain accumulation. When your only goal is plaque removal on a tooth or restoration that exhibits no stain and still has its luster, polish with a gentle toothpaste and a slow-speed handpiece or soft manual toothbrush.

Aluminum oxide paste can be used on composite resins, gold, and tooth structure. Begin to polish with extra-fine composite paste in a wet environment for best results. Remember to continually add water to the buffing cup. Distribute polish adequately over the entire surface and use a light intermittent stroke, contacting the restorative/tooth surface for no more than 15 to 30 seconds each. *The goal is restoration renewal—not recontouring or margin obliteration.* Carry paste interproximally with floss and rinse to clear area before re-examining.

If stain removal is the goal, and a paste alone does not achieve the desired results, it may be necessary to move on to more aggressive techniques in a logical manner.

Tools include varying paste grits, rotary rubber polishing instruments, and strips (in grades ranging from extra-fine through coarse). Rinse away the polishing agents and particles from the teeth or restoration, as well as the buffing cup, between levels of coarseness in order to avoid continually abrading the surface. Once stain removal is achieved, the final stage should be reversing the process and finish polishing with the least abrasive polish and instrument. This final step helps ensure that the surface texture is smooth and decreases surface energy. At the conclusion of each aesthetic management session, place a composite sealant over the definitive restorations and administer a neutral sodium fluoride tray application.

Porcelain and ceramic—as long as glazed or properly polished prior to seating— keep their gloss indefinitely. Polish only with an aluminum oxide paste on porcelain and ceramic restorations when resin cement or cementum is exposed. If the gloss is gone and only porcelain or ceramic is exposed, use a diamond polishing paste on felt wheels or a Robinson wheel. Diamond paste is best utilized in a dry environment, so use of cotton rolls, dry angles, or bite block is essential. With the appropriate polishing system, follow the same protocol and instrument sequence as outlined previously. But, a caution: Porcelain and ceramic materials may never return to their optimum gloss when polishing intra-orally.

Interproximal stain removal can be universally achieved with aluminum oxide polishing strips. Start with the finest grade and graduate to the next coarsest grade until the stain is gone. Complete the process by reversing the sequence and graduate to the finest grade until the restoration is smooth.

What clinicians must also keep in mind is that some of these treatments may never have the same luster they had the day they were placed. In fact—depending on the material used—they may actually appear aesthetically unpleasing, even after appropriate renewing and polishing techniques, though all are still functional. In other instances, the restoration may require replacing. Effective hygiene management starts when the difference can be assessed.

It is my wish that as we begin to gain knowledge in aesthetic renewal, we do not lose sight of a most important attribute: *education*. Do not incorporate any aesthetic-management session (such as new protocol, technique, and/or product) without first educating—both yourself and your patient—on the why, what, and how. Knowledge grows when shared and grows when used. Polishing procedures are not meant to be practiced silently.

For instance, explain to your patients why the new polish is more compatible with their dentistry. Let them know that, from now on, the polishing part will no longer feel like a sandy beach in their mouths. Polishing services need to be valued by the patient. You can do that by making them aware that such procedures can keep their aesthetic restorations looking their best for as long as possible. Delivering aesthetic hygiene excellence needs to equal creating and sharing team excellence.

Follow up Cosmetic Care with Vigorous 'Maintenance' Hygiene Appointments

By Lynn Miller, RDH
RDH Magazine, 1993, March; 13 (3): 42,44

Aesthetic hygiene management is not new; in fact, take a historical look back at the following article published almost 10 years ago. Granted—some of the terminology has changed and the product offering has increased, but excellence in hygiene is, what excellence in hygiene does!

Whether it is treatment acceptance, maintenance visits, or home health care, any dentist or hygienist has the greatest success with patient compliance when they reinforce benefits of the recommended procedure.

Refrain from going into great detail about the technical results or scientific studies that show why the patient should do what they need to do. Instead, emphasize that by proper maintenance, the procedure will last longer, heal properly, and look much better. (Occasionally, engineers, scientists, lawyers, or academicians love the scientific studies, so use them when applicable.)

Often, factual benefits are not as motivating as emotional benefits. These emotional benefits include how the patient will feel and look with your recommendation.

The endurance test for successful, functional, and esthetic longevity of any periodontal/cosmetic restoration is the dental office's maintenance procedures. Knowing *how* to identify early problems, curette, polish, and instruct the patient van be a wonderful source of comfort to the patient and a wonderful practice builder. Let your patients know you are specially trained in caring for the delicate procedures they have received.

Recall recommendations

Proper maintenance of the periodontally and cosmetically restored teeth can be one of the most vital aspects of the ultimate success of these treatments.

The long-term success of any periodontal and cosmetic procedure is the frequency and efficacy of prophylaxis, office care, and home care. The six-month "recall" appointment is *passé* with any type of implant, periodontal procedure, or cosmetic rehabilitation.

Three- to four-month prophylaxis appointments are mandatory. This should be emphasized before the patient accepts any periodontal or cosmetic treatment.

Label patients' charts with alert stickers that clearly proclaim "Periodontal Surgery," "Implants," "Porcelain Veneer," or "Bonded Veneer." Innovative Dental Concepts supplies stickers for such purposes.

This instantly reminds the entire staff that this patient needs to have a prophylaxis and recare appointment more frequently.

Restoration polishing and treatment

Porcelain veneers should be polished with diamond polishing paste, unless there is resin cement or cementum exposed. If either of the latter conditions exists, polish porcelain veneers with aluminum oxide polishing paste.

Diamond polishing paste, as recommended with porcelain, scratches and ditches cementum and resin cement. Composite veneers should be polished with aluminum oxide paste. Aluminum oxide polishing paste is safe to use on composites or porcelain.

During a prophy, any restoration with porcelain or composite material should be treated with sodium fluoride. For patients with root sensitivity or a high caries rate, frequent home use of sodium fluoride is indicated. Acidulated phosphate fluoride, on the other hand, can etch porcelain and composites.

Re-evaluation appointment

When patients present bleeding and inflamed tissue at their routine maintenance visit, scale and root plane the affected area and ask to see the patient again in two to three weeks. Even patients with moderate to severe gingivitis will need a re-evaluation appointment to ensure that the edema and bleeding have subsided.

Too often, hygienists assume a thorough prophylaxis, scaling, and root planing will remedy any infected tissue. It is no longer the standard of care to "cross your fingers" and assume the technique successfully treated the problem.

If the tissue is healthy at the re-evaluation appointment, shorten the patient's maintenance visit by one month. For example, if the patient is on a four-month recare appointment, shorten this routine to three months. If the tissue is not healthy and the bleeding persists, a thorough scaling and root planing per quadrant (ADA Code 431) or a referral to a periodontists might be necessary.

Reiterate the need for excellent oral hygiene for the maximum longevity of the restorations and periodontal health. A re-evaluation appointment is also necessary for patients with poor oral hygiene habits with or without gingivitis, since plaque may cause accelerated deterioration of cosmetic restorations and periodontal procedures.

If the gingivitis is persistent, check for overhanging margins on already places restorations, plaque level, and oral hygiene skills. Metabolic disruptions, such as medication, viruses, diabetes, and hormonal changes can all contribute to gingivitis.

Patient's home care

Oral hygiene skills need to be at their maximum before recommending Oral hygiene skills need to be at their maximum before recommending periodontal procedures or cosmetic restorations. A plaque-free environment is essential for the healing and maintenance of tissue.

Chart plaque indices and document all oral hygiene instructions in the patient's chart. An ultra-soft toothbrush is recommended for all cosmetic restorations to minimize scratching or abrasion.

Flossing becomes even more important, due to the harmful effects of plaque and acid on the proximal surfaces of composite or porcelain restorations. The use of a RotaDent (Prodentec) is also advised.

Home care of implants

Optimum home care is essential in maintaining the perimucoseal seal at the gingival/implant junction. The use of inter-dental brushes (Proxabrush, Oral B Inter-dental Brush) or a rotary uni-tufted brush (RotaDent) effectively removes plaque without harming the titanium abutment.

These devices also ensure that the margin of the prosthesis is not scratched. RotaDent's small soft brushes allow access to all tooth surfaces, including subgingival, ensuring a plaque-free environment with stimulation to the tissue.

In the case of hand brushes, make sure the bristles are coated with plastic or Teflon, preventing trauma to the prosthesis and soft tissue.

A patient with implants should be kept on a daily rinse of Peridex (chlorhexidine gluconate, .12%). It is advisable to have the patient dip the Proxabrush or RotaDent tips in the Peridex solution before cleaning around the implant.

Since chlorhexidine has the side effect of staining the prosthesis and other porcelain and composite restorations, it is advised to have the Proxabrush or a cotton Q-Tip dipped in the anti-microbial and applied to the site.

Educate patients during each visit

Patients should be educated about the needs three times in order to process what they need and what you are recommending.

We must next remember to go through the educational process of their dental needs each time we see the patient. The educational process might need to be a little different each visit, depending on how the patient is responding and reacting at that time.

And, finally, in the words of Omer Reed, "People don't care how much you know until they know how much you care." Basically, that means listening to our patient—first as a person, then as a patient. After carefully listening, we can take the patient to the next level for his or her dental treatment, maintenance needs, and home care.

If you do this process by listening, understanding, and loving first, you will almost instinctively know how to structure the conversation.

When your patients receive your knowledge—because they know you truly understand and care for them—you will get a much higher acceptance rate for whatever recommendations they need.

Dental Art Preservation

Step One: Understanding the rationale for esthetic/restorative management and renewal service

- Improves gingival health, less plaque retention

- Improves the compatibility of restorative material and oral soft tissues

- Increase the integrity of interface between restoration and tooth structure

- Improves cleansing by the patient

- Increases length of service of the restoration

- Establishes practice commitment to wanting dentistry to last

- Provides patients with a "renewed brightness"

- Expands service for hygienist and possibly certified dental assistants

Step Two: Identify

Clinicians must first differentiate natural tooth structure and the type of restorations.

- Mirco-hybrid, hybrid, microfill, porcelain, ceramic, etc.

Step Three: Evaluate

Determine the extent of polishing necessary, renewing, or replacement. Checklist for evaluating definitive restorations:

- Plaque accumulation
- Calculus accumulation
- Color match/ discoloration
- Staining
- Loss of surface glaze
- Labial/ palatal restoration(s) margin(s) integrity
  - Intact margin
  - Visible crevice at margin, crack visible on transillumination, fracture present, debonded/lost, overcontour, secondary caries, marginal leakage, microcracks, overhangs, open margins, undercontour margins, overcontour margins, ditches, grooves, etc.

Step Four: Stain Removal

A. Plaque or light stain removal

- A tooth or restoration that exhibits little to no stain, and the only goal is minimal stain and or plaque removal, can be polished with non-abrasive toothpaste or composite paste on a conventional soft-webbed prophy cup, polishing points, cups, or bristles.

B. Medium to heavy stain removal:

- Begin to polish with extra-fine composite paste, in a wet environment.

- Distribute polish adequately over the entire surface and use a light intermittent stroke contacting the restorative/tooth surface for no more than 15- 30 seconds each. (The goal is restoration polishing, not recontouring or margin obliteration.)

- Carry paste interproximally with floss and rinse to clear area before re-examining.

- If stain removal and high shine, leaving the desired surface texture on, are the goals, and a paste alone did not achieve the desired results, then it may be necessary to move on to more aggressive techniques in a progressional process.

  - Selections include higher grit pastes, impregnated-rubber polishing instruments, cups, discs points, strips, carbide burs—all in grades ranging from extra-fine through coarse.

  - Rinse away the polishing agents/particles between the levels of coarseness in order to avoid continually abrading the surface.

Once stain removal is achieved, reverse the process and finish polishing with the least abrasive composite polish/instrument to achieve the desired high shine and surface texture. *Remember to continually add water to the buffing cup, point, or brush.*

C. Interproximal Stain

- Interproximal stain removal and surface preservation can be universally achieved with aluminum oxide polishing strips.

- Start at the "safety center" with the finest grade and graduate to the next coarsest grade until the stain is gone.

- Complete the process by reversing the sequence and graduate to the finest grade until the restoration is smooth.

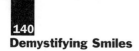

Step Five: Preserving composites

Stain at the margins, visual crevice, and/or "the little black line" that sometimes appears after placement may need additional care and renewal services.

Depending on state practice acts and allowable functions, determine the choice of instrumentation and product selection for this step.

- Severe microleakage/ open margins may require restoration replacement and a doctor's evaluation.

- Start with either a coarse point, diamond-impregnated rubber polishing points, slow-speed handpiece with a polishing/finishing bur, air abrasion (aluminum oxide), and or high-speed (carbide finishing bur, fissure prep bur.)

- Gently roughen the restoration to minimally open the margins and remove the irregular marginal staining and or "black line."

- Once the marginal stain is removed, scrub area clean by using a mixture of a cleaner/disinfectant and pumice with a brush applicator. Or use a chlorhexidine antibacterial scrub and a bristle brush in a slow-speed handpiece.

- Wash and dry the area.

- Etch the discrepancy several millimeters past the previously stained area. Use a disposable brush or applicator tip to agitate the etchant for 15-20 seconds. When renewing a composite restoration, the clinician may choose to use a plastic strip or guard interproximally to preserve the adjacent tooth.

- Rinse of the etchant for 5 seconds with an air-water spray

- Apply enamel-bonding agent.

- Apply the "renewal sealant composite material" from the syringe. A sable brush, small soft paintbrush, or applicator brush can be used to manipulate the renewal sealant.

- Cure "renewal sealant" for 40 seconds.

- Removal mylar strip/guard if used.

- Smooth/polish area with composite polishing paste.

Step Six: Increasing vitality and longevity

- Once either the stain removal procedures or the polishing services are complete, follow the final steps to further preserve the integrity of the restoration.

- Following polishing the restoration, use a disposable brush or applicator tip to agitate the etchant for 5 seconds. When applying a composite sealant, the clinician may choose to use a plastic strip or guard interproximally to preserve the adjacent tooth.

- Rinse the etchant for 5 seconds with an air-water spray.

- Dry

- Apply a composite surface sealant vigorously into the entire restoration, including margins with a mini brush tip.

- Gently blow off any excess.

- Cure the composite surface sealant for 20 seconds.

- Administer a tray/ neutral sodium fluoride application.

Sealant Insanity: My Road to Recovery

by Carol Jent, R.D.H., B.A.
Ultradent Products

So well I remember the early days of pit and fissure sealants. I recall envisioning happy, caries-free children and pleased parents thanking me for offering this revolutionary preventative service that would spare the child the drill and the parents the large bill.

Then the alarm woke me up.

The reality was that someone was asking me to make a six-year-old child sit still for a minimum of 30 minutes, while controlling their overly active tongue and trying to minimize a natural bodily function called salivating by stuffing cotton rolls in every corner of his or her mouth. If *that* wasn't enough, some dental manufacturer thought it would be easy to do all of this while dispensing drops of their A Resin and B Resin into a tiny reservoir, mixing and placing the resin with a dispenser designed by someone with too much time on their hands, and reaching for the curing light to polymerize the resin before it was contaminated by the saliva soaking through the cotton rolls.

Whew!

The final nail in the coffin was convincing the patient and the mom that I really had placed a preventative seal on the tooth, even though they couldn't see it.

Merely seeing the word sealants on the schedule during our morning huddle put me in a foul mood for the rest of the day. "No, it isn't a nice change of pace from gum gardening," I would tell the smirking doctor. "(This is still the case in a large majority of dental offices: The hygienist and assistant apply sealants.)

Many times, I would lower myself to offering large bribes to any one of my fellow co-workers in exchange for a helping hand with suctioning, holding the tongue out of the way, or just mixing the "Part A and B."

Of course, once the patient was out the door, it didn't end there. With each recare appointment, I found myself crossing my fingers and toes, hoping the sealant was still in place. When it wasn't, I blamed my own clinical skills.

Knowing there was no escape from what was touted a major step in preventative dentistry, I began a quest for the perfect sealant product.

The delivery system was my first area of consideration. Thankfully (and hopefully), the days of measuring and mixing resins from little bottles and dispensing uncontrollable phosphoric acid conditioner are gone. We now have products that are safe, premixed, and accurately delivered with syringes and tips that place the etchant and resins exactly where needed. Ultradent's UltraSeal XT Plus has a great delivery system. The InSpiral Brush Tip moves the resin through a helical channel where the resin is sheared to a thin consistency and applied with fine brush fibers. The resin placement is bubble-free and goes well into the deepest pits and fissures. The best part: Syringe-delivered materials can almost be placed with one hand tied behind your back—or, more importantly, with one hand holding cotton rolls, a saliva ejector, and a mouth mirror. (Figs. 5-1 through 5–5)

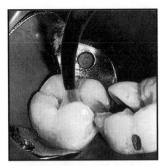

Fig. 5–1: *Cleaned and disinfected preparation, existing composite restoration, and occlusal grooves. Consepsis Scrub courtesy of Ultradent Products.*

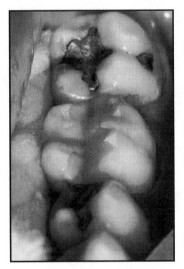

Fig. 5–2: *A clean existing composite restoration, courtesy of Ultradent Products.*

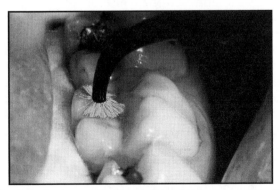

Fig. 5–3: *Brush composite sealant vigorously into surface. PermaSeal, Courtesy of Ultradent Products.*

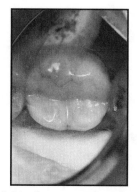

Fig. 5–4: *Four-year-old bonded Amelogen composite sealant, following a composite sealant treatment. PermaSeal, courtesy of Ultradent Products.*

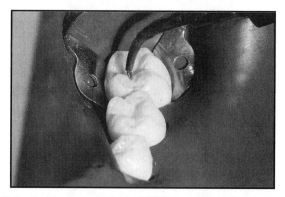

Fig. 5–5: *Applying sealant. UltraSeal XT Plus, courtesy of Ultradent Products.*

The second obstacle I was driven to overcome was "moisture contamination," the number-one cause of sealant failure. If moisture isn't dealt with on the first try, a second chance is almost a sure bet in about six months. To overcome such a threat, Ultradent includes (and highly recommends) PrimaDry in their sealant kits. PrimaDry is a drying and priming agent that requires 5 seconds to apply, but will save you a 30-minute reseal appointment later. Remember, the pits and fissures aren't empty spaces, and no matter how well you pumice the area, organic material will act as a sponge and hold water. Study after study has proven that using a drying/priming agent enhances the bond, the seal, and the longevity of the sealant.

Speaking of longevity: Find a product that is filled. Filled equals strength. Strength means its going to last. Because of the strength, highly filled sealant resins are also used as micro-restoratives and placed under composite restorations as a super-adaptive initial layer.

Fluoride-releasing sealants give the added bonus of protection. Many will release fluoride for a short time after placement, but quickly dwindle to nothing. There is now a natural fluoride on the market called FluorUtite, which is unique to Ultradent's UltraSeal XT Plus. Studies that compared FluorUtite to other leading sealants on the market found that it releases approximately twice the amount of protective fluoride at 52 weeks. (Fig.5–6)

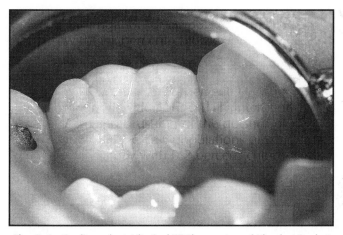

Fig. 5–6: *Quality sealant. UltraSeal XT Plus, courtesy of Ultradent Products.*

Many companies offer more than one shade of resin sealant, and clinicians have their reasons for choosing the one they use. Each shade has its own pros and cons. If you want the sealant to be seen when the patient goes out to show Mom in the waiting room, consider an opaque color. If you want the sealant to blend with the surrounding enamel shade, an A1 or A2 is usually the shade of choice. Clear or transparent shades were the first sealants to come to market and are still popular in many offices. With my trusty magnifiers, a good air syringe for desiccating the occlusal surface, and a sharp explorer, checking the sealants at recare is now not an issue.

Today, the industry is turning out more and better products, and the research is all pointing in a direction that says sealants are here to stay. I am a kinder, gentler, and more sane hygienist who appreciates happy, caries-free children and parents who thank me for offering this revolutionary preventative service that spares the child the drill and the parents the large bill.

Sealants

When dental sealants are accurately diagnosed and properly placed—and maintain seal—they work. As a preventive treatment modality, sealants can also greatly reduce dental care costs. However, proper pit and fissure assessment, placement modalities, or their management may escape many professional teams' clinical conscience.

First, let's clarify the varying descriptions and categories.

Traditionally, sealants have been successfully implemented in primary and secondary teeth for caries prevention. A sealant should sufficiently flow into the depth of the pit and fissures and completely bathe the spaces between etched enamel rods without covering the entire occlusal surface. The technique, though changing daily, must be carried out with complete isolation in a dry field, and the sealant must have continual management evaluations to ensure that the seal is retained.

Modern and conventional categories of sealants include:

- Composite/resin sealants
- Flowable resin-based composites (or preventive resin restorations—PRR)
- Unfilled sealants
- Filled sealants

Composite/resin sealants are specially formulated unfilled resins, designed to penetrate microcracks and/or defects after the finishing procedure of a newly-placed definitive restoration. They can prevent secondary caries by sealing restoration margins and the microcracks that may be responsible for wear, staining, and doorways for bacteria to invade the restoration/ tooth interface. Composite sealants wear, so re-application is necessary.

Flowable composites (or preventable resin restorations) are composite fillings diluted with unfilled resin material. The applications of preventable resin restorations are usually applied after carious lesions or suspicious stains are debrided from the pit and fissures. The rationale of opening up the grooves via a fissurotomy bur and or air abrasion (micro-dentistry) is that the carious process may be developing deeper in the fissure complex, below what a clinical explorer can detect. Current research questions the old hunt-for-the-stick-with-an-explorer or using X-rays (only about 25% accuracy) to determine the presence of a carious lesion. The theory here is that by the

> **Question:** *Want to make your clinical life easier?*
>
> **Strategy:** *Learn how to use a rubber dam*

time the radiolucency appears on a bitewing, the goal of minimal loss of healthy tooth structure has vanished. In response to the difficulties in assessing questionable occlusal caries, or to prevent the "W" word ("watch"), traditional assessment criteria can now be augmented to include newer available laser caries diagnostic tools and techniques.

Many contemporary sealants have filler particles included in their material, such as glass or quartz, to increase their resistance to wear and dissolution in the oral environment. Filler content can range from 20 percent to 60 percent. Filler particles will relate to a sealant's viscosity.

Other sealant properties to consider are shade (clinician's and patient's preference) and fluoride release.

Fluoride-releasing sealants add additional protection to surrounding tooth structures and have a potential for rechargeability after a fluoride application. In lieu of these data, the fluoride factor should play heavily in a clinician's decision when choosing a sealant product.

General steps for sealant placement

- Establish good illumination and magnification.
- Assess the tooth.
- Use explorer, appropriate radiographs, and/or laser caries identification machine.
- Clean the crevices with a prophyjet (air abrasion) or a cavity disinfectant and a stiff brush or a sharp explorer.
- Rinse the area out vigorously with air and water.
- Use a rubber dam, bite block, or dry angle.

- Follow the manufacturer's directions for etching time, primer, and sealant placement.

If a filler-particle sealant is used, it will not wear down easily, but should be inspected with articulating paper. Any overfilled areas need to be removed so as not to interfere with normal occlusion. At the completion of the service—as with any procedure that involves acid etches—apply a topical sodium fluoride.

Sealant management should include evaluation of retention. If a sealant falls out between hygiene sessions, the tooth needs to be re-evaluated before placing another sealant. In addition, if the sealant appears to be leaking or staining, caries-detection dye can be placed on the sealant. Using magnification, if a tint of the dye shows under the sealant, it confirms a leaking sealant. Caution should be exercised prior to resealing, to prevent the resealing of caries underneath.

Since filler particles incorporated in sealants are similar in structure (if not in percentage or weight) to the particles of composite restorations, sodium fluoride seems to be the fluoride of choice. Research involving glass ionomer cements, glass ionomer fillings, and composite restorations (both hybrid and microfill) shows acidulated phosphate and stannous fluoride increasing surface roughness and causing increasing restorative degradation and wear. Neutral fluorides and varnish appear to have no effect. Admittedly, these papers are based on studies performed mainly *in vitro* and on composite restorations, but one can draw comparable conclusions in regard to sealants. Potential and cumulative effects on the integrity of the sealant and its filler content must be carefully considered. If the surface becomes rougher, microorganisms could colonize at a faster rate, which would further affect retention.

Tooth Whitening

Tooth whitening can be traced to Biblical times. It was first documented in the dental literature around 1872, using oxalic acid to lighten non-vital teeth. In-office bleaching with hydrogen peroxide has been an accepted technique for more than 30 years. In addition, there are volumes of researched information and anecdotal validation that support the viability, safety, and effectiveness of professionally supervised 10 percent carbimide, take-home tooth whitening.

How it works

The two major players in whitening are carbimide peroxide (CP) and hydrogen peroxide (HP), with oxidation as the mode of action. Oxidation occurs when oxygen combines with stain molecules (chromagens) in enamel and dentin to make organic stains more soluble or invisible. The oxidation penetrates both enamel and dentin to remove organic material within the tubial structures and is dissolved into the saliva and oral environment. The results are notable changes in the refractory index of the enamel, lighter color at the dentinal level, opaqueness of the enamel layer, and teeth that appear whiter and brighter.

CP, a sustained release agent, whitens by breaking down into urea and hydrogen peroxide. These substances are well tolerated and excised by the body. CP has a slower rate of reaction than hydrogen peroxide. CP delivery usually occurs via a custom-made tray, worn between two hours and overnight. CP products are available in concentrations ranging from 10 percent to 30 percent.

HP, an immediate-release agent, breaks down into water and oxygen, often accelerated by enzymes such as peroxidase. Hydrogen peroxide releases oxygen within the first few seconds of contacting tooth surfaces, and its substantiality can last up to 30 minutes. HP products can be incorporated into tray whitening strategies if the patient desires a limited wear-time or prefers to whiten during the day: trays are typically worn two times a day for 30 minutes in addition to in-office power procedures. HP products come in concentrations of 5.5 percent and 7.5 percent.

Safety and efficacy

In 1994, the American Dental Association's Council on Dental Therapeutics published criteria for whitening in *Acceptance Program for Home-Use Tooth Whitening Products*. The guidelines were intended to document safety and efficacy. Before gels can be awarded with the ADA Seal of Acceptance, the program requires manufacturers to determine the degradation of bleaching gels in trays during use. In order for the whitening gel to be judged efficacious, the guidelines specify that results must indicate a tooth shade change of at least two shades according to a value-oriented Vita shade guide.

Abundant research documented since the early 1990s, plus thousands of successfully completed clinical cases, all point to authenticity of the safety and efficacy claims. In terms of safety, the research concludes that HP up to 3 percent and CP up to10 percent is non-carcinogenic. Many studies continually monitor negative effects that whitening has on tooth structure, pulp, and restorations, but no definitive conclusions have been determined as to long-term negative or irreversible results, in regard to the 10 percent CP formulations.

Whitening options

The hygiene assessment phase for new or current patients is the optimum time to begin educating and offering patients whitening procedures. Depending on what services your practice provides, some combinations include:

- Power whitening only
- Home whitening only
- Power whitening plus home whitening
- Laser whitening

Whitening strategy

The ingredient glycerin "dries" the tooth by leaching water from it. It can almost be thought of as a dehydrator agent. Earlier generations of whitening products used glycerin as a primary active agent. However, many manufacturers soon made the shift to glycol or water, once they found them to be less of a dehydrator. Check ingredients.

The whitening procedure should cease at least two weeks (10-14 days) before placing or replacing composites, veneers, or crowns in order to achieve a seamless match between definitive restoration and the new tooth color. This generally accepted time frame allows for complete color stabilization and hydration of the tooth structure.

After completing appropriate dental hygiene procedures, determine the pretreatment shade using a shade guide, and record it on the patient chart. Take pretreatment photos prior to delivering the whitening trays and post-treatment photos following the whitening treatment. In determining a personalized whitening option and agent, the clinician must identify the patient's preference for overnight or daytime whitening, or if he or she desires instant whitening gratification. Clinicians need to thoroughly explain whitening services and guide the patient toward the most appropriate method.

Patients need to understand that whitening is never 100-percent guaranteed, and that observed tooth color change can be dependent on some basic factors

- Whitening service
- Whitening time
- Initial tooth color
- Specific tooth region
- Etiology of stain
- Whitening product (concentration)
- Accuracy of tray fabrication
- Number of applications (laser and power)

Power whitening

Products in this category are usually 30 to 35 percent hydrogen peroxide. Some manufacturers recommend activating the whitening gel with a specialized curing light; others feel that a light source is unnecessary to activate the gel and/or will only expose the teeth to additional heat. While most clinical trials show that lights may have little or no effect on efficacy, many power gels have proprietary ingredients that require lights. It is difficult to set up comparison research studies to indicate which mode of action is superior and/or how effective a specific light spectrum is in enhancing the whitening process. With the increase in products available in this category, dental professionals must use their degreed knowledge to separate the glitz and promotions from safety and efficacy data.

Caution: Due to their high chemical concentrations, these whitening agents have a potential to cause significant soft tissue irritation and/or damage. Many manufacturers incorporate fluoride ions and or potassium nitrate to help minimize or eliminate sensitivity,

A properly placed and sealed rubber dam or a light-cured resin for soft tissue protection each provide appropriate barriers. Many office protocols include from one to three whitening sessions with 30 to 60 minutes contact time for whitening. Because some manufacturers recommend agitation of the bleach while on the teeth, team members need to be available so that the patient is not left alone with active gel on his or her teeth. Considerations for set-up, break-down, patient education needs, and team member or doctor supervision all need to be incorporated into the total chair time and fee.

Laser-assisted tooth whitening

"Laser whitening" as used in this section refers to professionally controlled, in-office services using a high concentration of hydrogen peroxide and an added energy source to excite the process of tooth whitening. Laser whitening is believed to accelerate the hydrogen particles to enhance whitening results. Laser whitening under the class II laser certification may require additional training and certification.

A handful of laser manufactures have received FDA clearance to use laser energy to whiten teeth. Their lasers are easily switched from a periodontal therapy instrument to a laser smile-whitening instrument by simply removing the soft tissue hand piece and replacing it with the whitening wand.

The caustic nature of the hydrogen peroxide precludes that the soft-tissue has suitable protection. A properly-placed rubber dam or a protective light-cured resin on the soft tissue provides appropriate barriers. These products are usually pre-mixed and are dispensed directly from their syringes onto the teeth.

A few additional safety concerns for both the practitioner and client include—

- Laser safety eye protection for everyone in the operatory
- First aid kit containing vitamin E, aloe vera, zinc oxide, and/or propylene glycol
- Extra concerns based on each individual patient's assessment and need

Further research is needed on laser whitening. Specifically, when choosing a suitable laser source, areas for the clinician to research include the efficacy of each laser and its wavelength, thermal effects of lasers, and pulpal response. Without compromise, follow the proper clinical protocol for the safety of the client and user.

Begin by discovering your patient's interest and goals for his/her aesthetic smile. Then, clinically review the patient's health and medical history to identify contra-indications for tooth whitening, such as pregnancy or nursing. It is also important to determine if the patient has used or is currently using any over-the-counter whitening products. We need to make sure the teeth will not be doubly treated! Be sure to document the product, brand, and patient usage. It is equally valuable to assess the patient's level of interest in advanced smile-enhancing procedures.

Before any whitening treatment is recommended, a complete clinical examination should be performed, including radiographs (to evaluate pulp chamber size). Intraoral examination of the teeth and soft tissues determines periodontal status. Decay, calculus, and extrinsic stains should be absent from the patient's teeth before beginning treatment. If any signs of disease are present, dental hygiene services or basic restorative procedures will need to be performed prior to the whitening regime. *It is strongly recommended that any patient interested in initiating whitening procedures first receive full preventive and therapeutic dental hygiene care.*

Additional considerations—such as recession and or TMJ dysfunction—should be discussed with the patient prior to initiating a whitening program. Recessed areas do not whiten as well and may also be more sensitive during procedures. Also, before beginning treatment, the patient should be made aware that existing tooth-colored restorations may not match the lighter shade of teeth after treatment and, as a result, may need to be replaced.

Home whitening

The professionally supervised home tray method has proven to be the most accessible and acceptable option for the majority of our patients' needs. It treats all the surfaces of the teeth and may be more advantageous in delivering low concentrations over a longer time period vs. intermittent high doses.

As mentioned earlier, these products contain various percentages of CP or HP. Other differences include viscosity, flavor, packaging, and whitening-tray material. During the oxidation process, the whitening agent demineralizes enamel rods from the enamel surface— right down to the dentin (and some studies have found the agent in the pulp chamber.) This process allows the bleach to directly contact and oxidize some of the chromogenic organic material in the underlying dentin. Now, assuming that a patient is given clear and understandable instructions, and does the home whitening correctly, enamel channels gradually open and remain open for the regimes, allowing greater contact with, and possibly a more profound effect, on the underlying dentin. Then, when a patient discontinues home bleaching, the more oxidized channels remineralize and close.

In the patient's record, remember to record the type of whitening gel used (CP or HP), the percentage dispensed to the patient (10 percent, 16 percent, or 22 percent), and the amount of gel dispensed.

Accurate tray fabrication will lead to more comfortably fitting trays and increase desired whitening results. Depending on manufacturers, tray fabrication and the inclusion, or not, of reservoirs (a thin layer of block out material placed on the facials of the teeth on the model before making the tray) continue to have their day on the debate floor. With reservoirs or without, the greatest importance is a comfortable, good-fitting tray.

The dental professional should also assist the patient as he or she practices placing the gel in the whitening tray and observe oral insertion. Overfilling of the guard could cause loss of material physically, whereas underfilling could cause voids that would reduce the duration of contact time between the agent and the tooth structure. Education should be verbal and written. The patient should be given a well-drafted and easy-to-follow handout. Instructions may include:

- Emphasis on effectively removing plaque and bacteria from the surfaces and between teeth before inserting the whitening tray.

- The use of a non-abrasive whitening dentifrice before, during, and after the whitening regime is completed to help fortify the achieved cosmetic results.

- Remove excess whitening material that may migrate on to gingival tissue after placement of the tray.

- Cease smoking and/or drinking of any dark-pigmented liquids during the process, and minimize the habits after completion.

- Contact the office if mild tooth sensitivity or gum irritation occurs.

- Schedule a follow-up visit one to two weeks after receiving the whitening kit to share concerns and successes.

Results can be observed within one to two weeks, and many patients report visible results within three days. Whitening evaluations completed by team members will further champion the profession's ability to develop patient-centered assessments and treatment planning. Many offices have found that whitening is the path for many patients to move into aesthetic/restorative procedures. In addition, it is vital to recognize the potential for increasing practice production through whitening.

- Consider that on average, a hygienist may treat eight patients a day.

- Assume, conservatively, that one patient per day chooses whitening.

- Multiply the number of days of the week the office works by the number of patients to achieve your potential for whitening.

- Plug your fees and "guesstimates" into this whitening formula to calculate your additional income potential.

- For instance: A practice sees patients four days a week and one patient per day chooses whitening. 4 x 1=4; 4 x 4 weeks per month = 16 x 12 months = 192 patients. Potential for power whitening (assuming a $700 total fee) = $134,400. Potential for home whitening (assuming a $500 fee) = $96,000

Remember, guessing is great, but tracking the actual dollars and case success rate is the "proof in the pudding" when it comes time for performance reviews!

Update on vital whitening

Practitioners have been aware that whitening teeth with tooth-colored restorations can create a shade difference between the new tooth color and the original restoration. The common thought is that the teeth change color while the restoration does not. Some studies are concluding that color changes *do* occur in tooth-colored restorations. More research is needed to establish a protocol to be able to accurately determine to what degree the restoration will change color; in the meantime, we must discuss this possible result with our patients prior to beginning whitening procedures.

Historically, HP solutions have been used to treat gingival inflammation. HP and CP are also documented as effective antimicrobial agents. One study, by Carolyn D. Bentley, D.D.S., concluded that a medium-viscosity 10 percent CP solution used in a fitted tray for only one hour per day for six weeks reduces lactobacilli (caries-producing bacteria) salivary levels. This means that some of the secondary benefits of whitening—at least during the whitening process and shortly afterward—may support a caries-control preventive plan.

A small amount of *in vitro* research has concluded that whitening agents chemically diffuse into the pulp chamber of natural and restored teeth. The degree of penetration into the pulp varies, depending on the whitening gels and pulpal chamber. In addition, diffusion varies, depending on restorative materials; for instance, composite resin material shows the least pulpal penetration. This information should be considered when developing whitening programs and explained to patients prior to whitening.

We are all familiar with the information that tetracycline causes discoloration of developing teeth in children. However, minocycline (sometimes prescribed for the treatment of acne and rheumatoid arthritis) also has the potential of causing pigmentations of teeth in the permanent dentition. The literature does not show conclusive or in-depth evidence as to the why, how, or when in the antibiotic treatment cycle this occurs, but it does suggest that a corresponding protocol of vitamin C may help prevent the discoloration.

Creating the whitening reservoir involves light-curing composite spacers on the patient's model prior to tray fabrication. These areas provide additional space between the tray and the teeth being treated. Recent studies have concluded that reservoirs are not needed for whitening to occur, and may not affect the clinical rate that whitening occurs or the efficacy of the whitening gel. Follow the manufacturer's recommendations.

Natural teeth will only lighten to a certain point/shade. Part of the pre-diagnosis is to record the shade prior to beginning treatment. During all follow-up sessions in the prescribed regimen, the shade of the teeth should be documented. This will aid in the final decision to stop treatment. If the teeth do not get lighter, the process should stop. After between three and seven days post-whitening, the patient should return for assessment and recording of the final shade and then move into the whitening-management phase.

White wall

...or, there is nowhere further to go with this type of service. And if our patients desire more, then we need to reformulate an appropriate treatment plan after a comprehensive dental hygiene prediagnosis and dental diagnosis.

If the patient's perception of optimal whitening has not occurred, further discussions about appropriate clinical services can be held. If the patient is happy, then at the beginning of every hygiene or restorative session, the shade of the teeth should be recorded. This will continue to add value to the original whitening process and alert both the professional and the patient if any color relapse has occurred. This monitoring will support timely and controlled touch ups. Remember, over-whitening will not induce further lightening and may lead to increased sensitivity, dehydration of the tooth structure, and reduction in enamel fracture toughness.

Create Your Strategies

Chance favors the prepared mind. • **Longfellow**

This exercise, provided at the end of each chapter, will assist you in designing a game plan in order to develop the skills, knowledge, and expertise necessary to propel you to your next level of personal and professional growth. Ask, answer, and record:

My smile-preserving care-delivery goals for the future are:

_____

_____

_____

The areas for which I would like assistance and support to achieve my goals are:

_____

_____

_____

My action steps to get in the game and achieve those goals are:

_____

_____

_____

My list of specific goals and dates I wish to accomplish them includes:

_____

_____

_____

Possible obstacles to watch out for (*i.e.,* fear of rejection, fear of change, and lack of accountability, denial, lack of focus, lack of self-evaluation, lack of mentoring relationships):

_____

_____

_____

Section III

Team Antics

SIX

The Big Game: Are You Ready to be Called Up?

The most important single ingredient in the formula of success is knowing how to get along with people. • **Theodore Roosevelt**

The New Breed of Hygiene Assistant
by Vicki McMannus, R.D.H.

Part I: Incorporating Team Hygiene

Hygiene mastery

If you've ever considered incorporating a hygiene assistant into your department, now is the time! The new breed of hygiene assistant is administratively savvy, clinically-oriented, and holds a high standard of care.

There are some huge differences between assisted hygiene and assisted suicide. Perhaps the thought of working out of two rooms with an assistant is a bit intimidating. You may be afraid of losing patient contact time or that patient education may suffer. Properly implemented, just the opposite occurs: You actually *gain* time with the patient, and the level of education is phenomenal.

There are a few basics to consider prior to beginning hygiene co-therapy. First, consider your own fears, and create a training program to address each of these. Next, incorporate the entire team in the transition from single-booked (on your own) hygiene to team hygiene.

Step one: Preparation

Your objective is to be a master at enrollment and have systems functioning at a high level prior to delegation.

1. Review and refine each system relating to the hygiene department. Recare, reactivation, diagnostics, examination, and educational protocols must be solidly in place prior to delegating tasks to others.

2. Create a "vision" with the doctor so that everyone is clear about the outcomes.

3. Identify the coordinator. Remember, her or his job is to make your schedule flow, enroll patients in care, and take on some of your duties. This has to be a high-caliber person. First, look within the practice. Is there a restorative assistant looking for more variety in her or his day, or an administrator who is looking for more clinical contact time? These are excellent candidates.

Jill Stedman of Tampa, Florida, is an excellent example of a high-caliber hygiene co-therapist. With more than 21 years of experience as a clinical chairside assistant, Jill was looking for more. In her own words, "I'd become burned out on making temporaries and taking impressions. I needed to connect with the patients on a different level. I was at the point that I was going to make a switch or get out of dentistry completely. Working in the hygiene department created a new challenge, one that I can see myself enjoying for many years to come."

Jill works with Deborah O'Shea, R.D.H. Together, this dynamic duo produces more than $350,000 per year working about 36 hours per week. Now *that's* productive! The best part for Deborah is a newfound freedom to concentrate on those aspects of hygiene that set her apart as a therapist. She now has the time to provide periodontal therapy at a high level, knowing that Jill is taking care of her schedule and providing incredible reinforcement and patient education.

Step two: Training–administratively

Your objective is to have your coordinator take on full accountability for the production of the department. This will necessitate an understanding of yearly, monthly, and daily goals as well as impeccable preferred status lists (also known as short-call lists) and confirmation protocols.

1. Review goal setting, scheduling, recare system, reactivation, and chart audit protocols with the coordinator.

2. Have the coordinator track daily production and look ahead to see if you are on course for the month.

3. He or she must have full understanding of charting and documentation. The coordinator can review charts each day for tomorrow's schedule and should have charts available when making the day-before courtesy call.

4. Clearly identify treatment needs and communicate this to the hygiene team. If bringing on an experienced clinical assistant is not possible in your office, consider an administrator who is looking to expand horizons.

Jackie Sullivan of Enfield, Connecticut, did just that. She was the recare secretary in a growing practice for more than 18 years when she decided to take radiation certification classes. From there, she started "hanging out" with the assistants and hygienists more. She has now blossomed into a world-class coordinator, managing a three-operatory hygiene department that is on the verge of becoming a million-dollar practice within the general dental practice—again, working a four-day work week!

Jackie says, "The key to delegation is building trust. The hygienists have to know that I will take care of their patients in the same manner they would. Otherwise, the whole system falls apart. I am one part air-traffic controller and one part patient advocate. I can socialize with the patients in the reception area so the patient is more relaxed and comfortable before we even begin the appointment. I make the day flow, and I love it!"

Step three: Training–clinical

Your objective is to have a highly skilled, well-trained professional on your hygiene team.

1. Take the time to train your assistant in the following areas. Her or his clinical skills, as well as a gentle approach, are critical.

   a. Medical history update (including blood pressure)

   b. Identifying dental concerns

   c. Intra-oral camera tour

   d. Radiography

   e. CAESY educational system

   f. Basic self-care instruction

   g. Periodontal and restorative recording

   h. Doctor examination protocol

2. Schedule a week of observation and gradual delegation on a single-booked schedule. Have the assistant shadow you and listen to your patient conversations for the first day.

3. Pay particular attention to communication scripts for:

   a. Greeting the patients and creating rapport

   b. Enrollment of x-rays, fluoride

   c. Enrollment of restorative and periodontal care

   d. Education regarding self-care

   e. Creating value for continuous care

   f. Handling financial objections

4. On the second day, continue with the single-booked schedule. Begin allowing the assistant to seat your patient and initiate the appointment. This is your time to watch your assistant. Remember, soon you will be in another room. Take this time to teach your assistant so that you will feel comfortable letting go of the patient.

5. You must develop trust with your assistant. Now is the time to do it.

6. Make note of all things she or he did well.

7. Make note of areas requiring improvement.

8. When you are comfortable with seating protocol, move on to medical history update, x-rays, and intra-oral camera tour.

9. By day three, you should be functioning well with your assistant in place on a single-booked schedule.

Jose Morey of Seattle, Washington, is paired with Amy Mitchell, R.D.H., and the hygiene team for Dr. Michael Koczarski. Again, she was once "discovered" from the doctor's clinical team. Her belief is that having a strong sense of the doctor's recommendations helps her to communicate with the patients. She can work with the hygienists to identify patient need and educate them to possible treatment modalities. This frees up valuable time for both the hygienist and the doctor.

Dr. Koscarski says, "Shifting Jose to the hygiene department took a big leap of faith. I didn't think that I could easily replace her on my side. The truth is, I didn't lose her, and she supported the training of our new assistant as she was transitioning into the hygiene department. She made it smoother for everyone. We all depend on her to blend the hygiene and doctor schedules and make our day work."

Hygienist, you are now ready to delegate to your assistant because you have developed the trust that she or he is giving your patient the same care you would.

Assistant, you now have an understanding of what your hygienist needs, and you operate from the belief that you can provide whatever she or he needs, whenever she or he needs it. This is the ultimate in patient care!

Part II—Incorporating Auxiliaries into the Hygiene Department

Helpful guidelines for assisted hygiene
- Start slow
  - Overlap only 10 minutes at the beginning and end of each appointment
  - Start with one to two days per week, work up from there
- Hire an individual who already knows your practice
  - ACE: attitude, communication, enthusiasm
  - Train for skill

- Get the team involved. What are the benefits to patients and practice?

- Provide written job descriptions

- Be flexible

- Keep a daily time table for one month

- Keep schedules for each day, including what worked and what didn't

- Schedule weekly hygiene meetings—forever

- Revaluate periodically

  - Increase time overlap to 20 minutes at the beginning and 20 minutes at the end of each appointment

  - Evaluate capacity on a quarterly basis—adjust templates

Part III—Job Descriptions

Hygiene assistant

The hygiene assistant functions as a "coach" for clinical staff, develops a game plan, and facilitates in the correct implementation of each play. The assistant supports hygienists in:

- Documentation and charting

- Scheduling and confirming appointments

- Taking radiographs

- Coronal polish (if allowed by state law)

- Patient education

- Setting up and breaking down rooms

- Setting up intra-oral imaging

- Entering treatment plans

- Placement of sealants/restorative materials (where permitted)

- Assistance with laser therapy

- Assistance in sterilization and infection control of the office

- Responsibility for chart auditing and internal marketing

- Creating a "priority list" of patients who can come in for treatment on short notice

- Ordering hygiene supplies

Hygiene coordinator

- Serves as the hygiene department leader

- Leads hygiene department meetings and serves as team leader for all staff meetings

- Functions as an advocate for discussions of concerns between hygienists and docto.

- Orders all hygiene-related instruments, brochures, supplies, and home-care aids

- Maintains and tracks inventory of all the above supplie.

- Facilitates the training of new hygiene staff members. Aids in training entire team on updated hygiene procedure.

- Aids the doctor in submitting new clinical information to the hygiene department

- Tracks upcoming continuing education courses

- Designs and implements ideal hygiene schedule

- Sets hygiene department goals and monitors. Responsible for tracking and submitting these monitors at staff meetings

The Treatment Plan You Always Wanted but Didn't Know You Needed

by Kathleen Johnson
Kathleen Johnson and Associates

Several weeks ago, as I was perusing the selection of sunglasses at a local store, I found myself eavesdropping. A young father had just wheeled his toddler into the children's aisle to choose a hat to protect her from the sun during their upcoming vacation. The child immediately became enthralled with a blue plastic sun visor stamped with the Little Mermaid, while the father's inclination was toward a purple canvas hat, brimmed all the way around. She fiercely shook her blonde curls in refusal as he pleaded about how the purple hat would protect her face and her back when they were on the river.

Although his choice cost a full $10 more, he looked at the price tag on the Disney visor and clicked his tongue. "$3.99," he claimed in mock horror. "Sweetie, that's so much money. I'm not sure Daddy can afford it." She responded with a look that said she already knew Daddy could afford anything she wanted.

In a final brilliant attempt, the father held the purple hat up wistfully and said, "It's just as well. Being purple and all, this is probably a princess hat. They may not have even let us buy it anyway." The girl immediately discarded the visor in favor of the purple princess hat, and they headed for the check out line.

The father knew his daughter *needed* the purple hat, and he knew she *wanted* the hat she believed was more special—more fairy tale. So, he helped her to *want* the hat that she truly *needed*.

The field of dentistry requires similar sales know-how. Many Americans do not value their oral health. While most people immediately accept the treatment recommended by medical doctors, they fail to complete (or refuse to even start) much of the treatment recommended by dentists. Like the little girl in the store, patients are more likely to accept the treatment they *want* rather than the one they *need*. Therefore, if dentists want to run successful practices and want to help their patients achieve oral health, they must present each treatment plan in a manner that makes the patient want the treatment they truly need.

Presenting the treatment plan

You've heard the old expression "Things will look better in the morning." But when we put things off, they really don't get better—they only *look* better. In reality, they often get a lot worse.

This is why the treatment plan must be presented in the treatment room immediately following the exam and diagnosis. At this point, both the assistant and the dentist should have familiarized the patient with the problem so he or she will feel a sense of urgency. Don't forget: Many patients unnecessarily fear dentistry, and this dread is something we are constantly working against. The patient is still seated in the chair at this point, and the dentist or hygienist can conveniently redirect the patient's attention to the problem and its consequences using mirrors, the computer screen, diagrams, or models while alleviating his or her fears over the procedure.

Deciding who presents the treatment plan

When I was a little girl and I asked my father for ice cream money or permission to play at a friend's house, he would say, "What does your mother say?" Not because he did not feel like he knew what was good for me, but rather because he needed to understand all the circumstances and he knew it was important, whatever the final decision, for he and my mother to maintain a common front. Divisiveness undermines authority.

The dentist must be the one to present the initial treatment plan; however, it is crucial that every member of the staff reiterate the same concerns and recommended solution throughout the patient's entire visit. In addition, it is a good idea to offer magazines, books, or videos that reinforce the diagnosis and the treatment plan.

Presenting the full treatment plan

A friend of mine recently purchased a new car. Her husband, who owns a construction company, was to be out of the state for nearly a month at a work site, and it became clear that they needed to purchase a new car before he left. Together they decided how much money they wanted to spend and transferred that amount from their savings to their checking account. At the import lot, the dealer, perhaps influenced by my friend's attire—always jeans and a T-shirt—tried to direct her attention to some of the less-expensive models. Once she became interested in one, he encouraged her to think about it a little longer and come back with her husband so that he could make a final decision.

Needless to say, she left the lot as he suggested, but she wrote a check, in full, for a more expensive car on another lot less than an hour later. The first car dealer lost her business because he made assumptions about what kind of car she could afford and how capable she was to make an important decision.

We must refrain from making these kinds of assumptions about our patients. Everyone deserves the same quality dental care. With every patient, we are working toward the same ideal of a healthy mouth and a confident smile.

Discussing financial arrangements

I have a house full of animals—two cats, two birds, and two dogs. I have found a good veterinarian, one who is gentle with my animals and with me; one who I know would never cheat me. When there is an emergency with one of my pets, I accept her diagnosis and treatment plan immediately, without questioning the cost. I know that she is fully competent and that her staff will help me formulate a financial plan before I leave.

This is the atmosphere we want to build in the dental office. The dentist should never discuss financial arrangements. If a patient feels pressure about finances, that pressure could affect the dentist's diagnosis as well as the patient's acceptance of the treatment plan, jeopardizing the patient's oral health. Instead, a financial coordinator or advisor (a staff member who has a caring demeanor and who is familiar with all insurance benefits and policies and third-party financing) must present a financial plan separate from the treatment plan presentation.

Ideally, this discussion should take place face-to-face in a quiet area where the patient and the financial coordinator can talk privately, and it should occur after the patient has already accepted treatment. This conversation should not center on whether or not the patient can afford the treatment, but rather *how* the patient can afford the treatment. The coordinator must recommend the optimum treatment, exploring other possibilities only at the patient's request. The dentist should also be prepared to address the kinds of behavior or neglect that have contributed to the problem, the specific degree of the current problem, and what consequences the patient can expect if the problem is allowed to progress further.

Maintaining healthy practices

Dentistry is not like microwaves, cell phones, or cappuccino—things we are introduced to and then think we cannot live without. Proper dental care is a necessity. Presenting it to your patients in a manner that will get them to respond, while important to the strength of your practice, is even more important to the health of your patients.

The Aesthetic Hygienist

by Deborah Dopson-Hartley, R.D.H.

The job description and responsibilities of the aesthetic hygienist are not the status quo. With the increasing demands made on us by expanded functions, indoctrination of aesthetic dentistry, implementation of consultants, incorporation of advanced continued education courses, managed care and insurance dilemmas, and ever-expanding state and federal regulations, we find there is more for us to do in the same amount of time—or, for production's sake, *less* time.

In order to thrive (let alone survive in today's changing health-care market), we all must be educating and re-educating, defining and redefining, and focusing and refocusing on our job descriptions, business strategies and plan, and simply how we do our jobs. Under-utilization of the hygienist, our education, our skills, and our time simply does not make good business sense.

Comprehensive restorative aesthetic dentistry is extremely technique-sensitive, and timing is everything. There is simply no room for error! For a comprehensive aesthetic practice to be truly successful, the doctor must have total concentration to perform this difficult and complex work. The aesthetic dentist simply cannot carry the burden of education, internal marketing, and motivation of comprehensive aesthetic dentistry for patients.

So, the aesthetic hygienist must help carry this burden. Hygiene now needs to not only mine the mother lode, but must also comb out the nuggets in the recare system. We must now become even more effective at internal marketing and become effective salespeople, as well. When we consider the fact that we spend more time with patients than any other person in the practice—doctor included—then we really owe it to the business to become the number-one educator for all types of dentistry, especially aesthetic.

With these thoughts in mind, here are some steps you can take to improve your ability to promote comprehensive restorative aesthetic dentistry and, ultimately, to bring a steady flow of cases to your practice.

In order to educate, motivate, and influence patients to pursue their dental wants and needs, hygienists must know how and why dentists do the things they do. How can we explain the treatment of a particular procedure that's been recommended if we don't truly understand it?

How can hygiene improve the patient's dental IQ without improving our own?

First, go beyond those basic, mandatory hygiene continuing-education requirements. Next, go to the seminars, study groups, and workshops that your doctor attends. Read their journals and newsletters and listen to their collection of tapes. During down time, watch or assist your doctor during procedures. By doing this, you will not only experience for yourselves the truly marvelous advances dentistry has made, but also understand the new level of commitment to this dentistry as well.

You will then have the same understanding, enthusiasm, and passion that dentists have. You will be able to transfer those same empowering emotions to the patients. As my own enthusiasm and passion towards aesthetic dentistry increases, so does patient acceptance.

The "dentist to the stars" (and my other boss), Dr. Larry Rosenthal, once said during our six-day hands-on program, "The eyes cannot see what the mind does not know. But once your mind knows, your eyes cannot help but see it every time." He was right.

With my new understanding of comprehensive aesthetic dentistry, I've become more confident and competent to really look at and discuss smile designs and reconstruction with our patients. I can now see what my comprehensive restorative aesthetic dentist sees. I can pre-diagnose, draw up treatment plans, and discuss with patients comprehensive care with near accuracy. I am comfortable with case representation because I understand the comprehensive restorative aesthetic concept. I now see every patient as a canvas.

But this level of dentistry is far more challenging to market. It requires a higher level of education, commitment, and time—lots of time. People don't always understand it. Everyone knows what crowns are, how expensive they are—and no one wants one. Few people know about inlays or veneers, but most know their insurance won't pay for it.

Helping patients understand this new technology—elevating and changing their value and belief system—will only help them make the right choices (and "so what" if insurance doesn't pay!). Patients need not feel pressured or sold on unwanted or unneeded services. Rather, they need to feel trust, support, understanding, and encouragement to be able to move forward with their dental-health needs and goals and act on their desire to improve their appearance and their overall dental health.

So, what is the true value of the aesthetic hygienist?

We do much more than just treat peoples' teeth. We help to restore their dignity. This is more than cosmetic dentistry. It's about esteem and helping people feel good about themselves. It's about restoring dignity thorough cosmetic dentistry

These are truly exciting times when it comes to all the wonderful aesthetic and dental services we can now offer patients. This is a new era, full of opportunities. Take this opportunity and turn that great potential into real treatment cases by recognizing and building on your true value as a hygienist and as a vital part of your practice's team. Educate yourself and become the type of hygienist your practice wants and needs. Become an aesthetic hygienist.

The Hygiene Treatment Coordinator: The Messenger

by Allison Roberts

What is a full-time hygiene treatment coordinator? What is an aesthetic hygienist? What is an aesthetic hygiene assistant? How is any of this an added benefit to the practice? I know— more overhead and yet another employee; sure, why not?

Are you confused? So was I.

I am the full-time hygiene treatment coordinator for aesthetic hygienist Deborah Dopson-Hartley, R.D.H.—a person I first met by reading about—and am an expanded-functions dental assistant for Dr. Diane Wright, an aesthetic dentist. Deborah taught me to convert traditional methods of hygiene into a very successful and rewarding program called T.E.A.M-HYGIENE—and I love it. I hope my story will open your eyes to the change and the possibilities that have made all the difference in my life and career.

As Deborah states in many of her articles, "Time is money, and under-utilization of our time, education, and expertise simply does not make good business sense." I guess we need to decide: Why are we here? My view is that we are here to provide efficient, comprehensive, and optimal patient care in a comfortable, serene environment. To be able to do this, we have to establish the most important thing: Trust.

Whether it is the new patient experience or just a follow-up maintenance appointment, building rapport with the patient is all part of a hygiene treatment coordinator's job. I am not here just to take x-rays and prep the patient so the hygienist can buy time. I am here to establish a relationship with patients and discuss their needs, wants, desires and, most of all, their problems and concerns. I educate and help motivate patients to say "yes" to the best.

In our office, Deborah has me polishing our patients first—wow! Now, *that's* different! Establish yourself as "different." Patients like that. We are not the norm. We cordially explain that we like to polish first so that we do not introduce any new bacteria into the bloodstream. Deborah likes to begin with a clean environment so that she and our dentist can better assess and evaluate the health status of the gingival tissue.

As I continue to polish the patient, I open my eyes to possibilities. I visualize my patients as an artist regards a canvas. What will the end result be? I ask open-ended questions and listen closely to the responses. Could this patient benefit from amalgam removal, cosmetics, or possible tooth replacement with either implant therapy or all-porcelain bridgework? Intra-oral photos, cosmetic imaging, and the CAESY education systems allow me to utilize my time as the hygiene treatment coordinator *productively*. I help with the periodontal charting and then kindly dismiss myself from the room to meet the next patient.

I sit in on the doctor's exam, as well. In my opinion, the exam is the most important part of the appointment. Since Deborah and I have gathered all the necessary information—periodontal chartings, areas of concern, intra-oral photos, x-rays, cosmetic imaging, chief complaints or concerns—it is now time for me to pass the baton. As "the messenger," communication is key: The hygiene treatment coordinator must effectively communicate all of the patient's concerns to the hygienist and the doctor to ensure quality of care. From a business perspective, no matter how much Deborah and I educate the patient, the doctor must confirm treatment or all that hard work and production walk out the door unscheduled.

After treatment and diagnosis, I schedule the next appointments, listening to and answering any questions. I can then dismiss a patient who is now fully informed of his or her needs and is excited about treatment. Trust is now established!

Ask for referrals. Give out your doctor's business cards. You'll be amazed at how many new patients will call.

Dentistry has so much to offer, and we take great pride in our staff's training and capabilities. Be dedicated to excellence; accept nothing less. As our new-patient welcome brochure says: "Welcome to total-quality dentistry, delivered with an unparalleled degree of personal respect, sincere friendship, and absolute professionalism."

It takes perseverance, passion, and pride in yourself and in what you are doing to succeed in life. My goal is to make a difference for at least one patient a day. Make them smile, understand, and know that they are cared for. Dr. Wright and Deborah Dopson-Hartley have given me the opportunity to make that difference.

What I have learned by being in charge of the hygiene department is just how challenging it is for hygienists to practice traditional hygiene. As Deborah has stated: "It just doesn't make business sense." My passion for dentistry has evolved and my insight into total patient care has broadened by being part of T.E.A.M.-HYGIENE and an aesthetic hygiene assistant.

Hygiene Business

Only a hygienist completely informed about the hygiene business and the numbers generated in his or her department can truly make the "I deserve it!" statement when it comes to compensation issues.

Why? Because only when you know and understand all the figures associated with running a profitable hygiene center, and how your daily, weekly, monthly, quarterly, and yearly profit-and-loss numbers align, can you determine how much money can be spent on upgrading a hygiene smile gallery.

Is the hygiene department profitable enough to reward the hygienist with an increase in compensation, or to buy the latest and greatest equipment? That's what hygienists must discover—and they can do so by assessing the hygiene department's bottom line and asking questions.

- Is hygiene production, compared to total office production, at least 30 percent?

- What are current and previous years' percentages of 1110s, 4341s, and/or 4910s?

- What are the percentages of adult topical fluorides, composite and preventive sealants, occlusal guards, home-service products, and whitening services?

- What is the percentage of successful pre-appointing of all hygiene patients?

- How much cosmetic/restorative treatment was prediagnosed in the hygiene department? Which procedures? What was the percentage of case acceptance—not just discussed, but actually scheduled and performed? (Fig. 6-1)

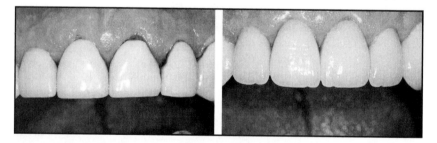

Fig. 6–1: *Before and after photos of anterior sextant, dentistry courtesy of J. Schmid, D.D.S.; lab work by Aurum Ceramic.*

Have you evaluated the percentages of cancellations and no shows, and calculated the crippling affect they have on your production numbers? For example, if the targeted hygiene production goal is $100 per hour and you have four hours open per week due to no-shows or cancellations, that equates to $400 in lost revenue. Continue this scenario over a month ($400 x four weeks) and the loss is $1,600. How about over the course of a year? This example does not even consider the overhead expenses that are still adding up while the chair is empty.

Can you now begin to see an area that may be taking away from your new equipment want list?

Be astute to the business information—take responsibility for the hygiene schedule—and hygienists can determine *for themselves* how much money is available for hygiene development (such as salaries, continuing education, and equipment). Currently, there are user-friendly management systems that can run daily reports so a hygienist can easily track the numbers. In addition, if numbers prove to be less than stellar, enlist the talents of a hygiene or practice coach who can guide the hygiene department (and, ultimately, the practice) to a higher level.

Many practices have daily hygiene goals. However, it is surprising to see how few hygienists know how to figure their *actual* daily average. To determine profitability and where the goal should be set, a hygienist must know her or his daily compensation (including benefits). One formula for determining profitability and goal is "the 3 X's":

Hygienist's Salary + Benefits = Goal

Hygiene is about discussing, facilitating, and managing the synergy of health, beauty, and function, and the hygiene department is a major part of the fuel that sustains a dental office. When hygienists are not providing ultimate preventive care, pre-diagnosing aesthetic and restorative cases, *and* tracking and evaluating the business data, the entire office engine could stall. This means "no" to purchasing new products or equipment and "no" to innovative hygiene services.

So, before creating your next hygiene "wish list," be sure you clearly understand the business aspect of the hygiene department. After all, that is what any CEO would do!

Break it down, before putting it back on the fast track

- Do you have a vision statement developed specifically for the hygiene department?

- Do you have a clearly defined clinical, non-surgical periodontal protocol and philosophy that each team member supports?

- How many bleeding points (on provocation) are acceptable to qualify a service as non-surgical therapy?

- How many bleeding points (on provocation) determine that a patient is now in the management phase of non-surgical periodontal therapy?

- Do you have a clear and defined pre-diagnostic aesthetic and restorative philosophy and protocol that each team member supports?

- Can you discover and communicate aesthetic and restorative possibilities? (Fig. 6–2)

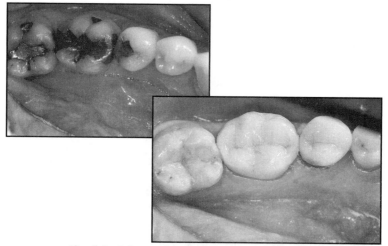

Fig. 6–2: *Before amalgam and after laboratory processes.*
Dentistry courtesy of Stephen Poss, D.D.S.; lab work by Aurum Ceramic.

- Have you established clear distinctions and categories for all hygiene department procedures, for example, you do not treat any periodontal condition as an 1110 prophy procedure?

- Do you utilize the intra-oral camera or digital photography?

- Are you confident that your clinical protocols and technology are state of the art, with evidence-based research?

- Do you have a protocol or someone accountable to establish what is working and what is not? (identifying treatment obstacles, technology opportunities, etc.)?

- Do you have a dedicated hygiene assistant?

- Do you engage patients in oral-health concerns?

- Do you have a seamless doctor/hygiene system that increases case acceptance?

- Do you have continuity among team members for all clinical, managerial, and behavioral procedures?

- What is your hourly goal?

- Do you have an agreed-upon daily production goal?

- Do you have access to such tracking information?

- Do you have daily monitoring systems for hygiene?

- Are you monitoring the number of procedures performed in hygiene (prophy, non-survival perio, sealants, adult fluoride, renewal and management of restorations, etc.)?

- Do you know how close your year-to-date percentage of hygiene production is to goal?

- What is your total year-to-date percentage hygiene production versus total office production?

- Do you have a low-opening percentage, per day, per hygiene schedule?

- Do you have management tracking systems in place to monitor pre-diagnosis case presentations and closures?

- How many active patients' charts are in your practice (seen within 18 months)?

- How many hygiene patients are scheduled per day?

- Do you consider dental hygiene a career?

- Break down the services: How many are for recare, perio, perio management, restorative management, sealants, whitening, etc.?

- What is the current year-to-date number of 1110, 4341, and 4910 procedures? Previous year ratios of same?

- What is yearly hygiene production? Compare that to last year.

- What is the total number of hygiene days worked? Compare that to last year.

- What is average daily production? Current year per day? Previous year per day?

- Do all recare patients get the same amount of time regardless of treatment needed?

- Do you utilize a customized time-management system for recare sessions?

- Do you perform chart audits?

- Do you pre-reserve patients for their next hygiene session?

If you don't know what to do with all this information, hire a reputable hygiene coach to support your move to the next level!

Educating Patients on the Value of Dental Investment/Dental Insurance Independence

How are fees and insurance issues addressed with your patients? How well do you feel that you can talk about fees?

Do you talk about fees openly and confidently with patients? If patients sense that any team member does not support the fee structure of the practice, the entire practice is undermined.

Do patients know it's okay to openly address these issues with you? How supportive do patients think you are about the subject of fees? How can this topic be addressed in the first inquiry call? How well do you address this topic in the office—in person or on paper? Is this topic addressed in printed material you offer about your practice?

Are you assisting patients with financial and insurance matters?

Insurance: Is it the bad guy?

Some offices do not try to judge a patient's insurance company as "good" or "bad." They have found that speaking negatively can reflect poorly on the practice. Insurance is just another financial tool for payment. It is nothing more than a contract to pay benefits. The decision is whether your practice decides to accept insurance assignments—or not. If it does, then the office must be prepared to handle the sweet and the sour.

Do You Say "My Way or the Highway?" (Tomato or To-motto?)

As a speaker, I often hear the woes of clinical hygienists who are frustrated with their employment homes. Many hygienists attempt to leave the prophy-mill offices for what they expect to be quality, value-added practices. Unfortunately, sometimes the only distinguishable differences between the old and the new are not standards of care or team relations, but in the décor, marketing material, and loss of faith!

Situation/overview from one hygienist

"I wanted a change and began work with an aesthetic dental office. I interviewed with the doctor, who was very impressed with my periodontal background.

"When I arrived to observe before my first clinical day, I immediately noted a strong office belief, almost cult-like, in a particular practice-management philosophy. Before I began, I had to watch videos, listen to audiotapes, and read numerous books in the art of selling dentistry. [*Many hygienists are open to theses new learning tools and even excited about what they are now being exposed to.*] They light candles and bake breads and cookies. Waterfall rock fountains are featured throughout the office, and they keep air fresheners in each operatory. [*Again, to this point, hygienists who tell the story still have a spark and passion for this new-age value dental environment*].

"Now, as I begin to work with patients, I am told that the previous hygienist only took about 15 minutes, total time, to perform hygiene services. The doctor tells me, "It is not about cleaning teeth, it is about building relationships."

"Patients do not know the difference as long as their teeth are smooth and polished. The doctor wants me to ask the patient, 'How do you like to have your teeth cleaned? Do you like to not know that I am in your mouth or do you like a really thorough job?' [*Now the storyteller's posture and speaking style begins to shift, taking on a more defeatist tone.*]

"In addition," she says, "Listen to what is expected of me in this front-deskless environment!"

- Take needed radiographs (FMX–24 double films)
- Full periodontal charting (once a year, with no assistant to help, and I have to enter the readings into the computer at a later time since there is no voice activation in the hygiene room)
- Reappoint the next recare session
- Post charges
- Collect payments (of course, there is no credit card machine in my operatory, so I need to go the to the front-deskless front desk")
- Post-treatment plan with the proper ADA codes (which I do not know, and so I have to always locate the master key sheet)
- Provide the necessary hygiene service
- Oral hygiene instruction
- Clean and disinfect hygiene room
- Order supplies
- Send equipment out for repairs
- Stock rooms
- Call two patients a day to "see how their appointment went"
- Write a card to one patient a day
- Ask for referrals
- Ask about long-term dental health goals for the next 20 years early in the appointment so that I can do a one-to-one interview
- Update meds, dental Rx
- Audit charts
- Change processor chemicals, ultrasonic cleaners
- Help everywhere I can since the office policy is "every job is everyone's job"

- Arrive 30 minutes prior to my first patient and do not leave until around 5:30 P.M., although I only get a salary for the hours of 8 A.M. TO 5 P.M.

- "We are supposed to receive bonuses 'after profit'; I was told they average $200 a month. After three months, I have yet to see any bonuses and I am unsure how that all works. If I were just paid for the time I was there, I would not *need* bonuses."

Finally, she concludes, "I am looking for other employment. I was disappointed in an aesthetic dental office."

It has been said that there are no bad people, just bad systems that good people are forced to endure every day. It appears that in many of these scenarios, the hygienist is looking for the perfect office, and the office has fallen victim to the "guru syndrome." This occurs when a doctor or team buys into everything and anything that a speaker or a practice-management consultant says or recommends. Then, upon coming home after a weekend conference, immediately abandons the old ways for the new ways without actually taking the time to evaluate what was working and what was not working in the practice.

There are so many opportunities in these scenarios for a hygienist (or any team member) who feels disconnected to attempt to reconnect and understand. Here, I offer some areas to explore before you decide to leave one office for another.

- Make sure you have clear expectations prior to accepting a job.

- Schedule a meeting with the doctor to explore possibilities—and speak up.

- Is there a written job description?

- Have someone explain the bonus system to you, and determine who is accountable for that information. Who can you go to, to find out why it is not paying out?

- What is the written nonsurgical periodontal program for the office?

- If the office is "front desk-less," will you have a dedicated hygiene assistant?

- What would you do to design your own game plan if you were the hygienist in this situation?

Create Your Strategies

Have patience with all things, but mostly with yourself. •**St. Francis DeSales**

This exercise, provided at the end of each chapter, is to assist you in designing a game plan in order to develop the skills, knowledge, and expertise necessary to propel you to your next level of personal and professional growth. Ask, answer, and record:

My goals for "the big game" for the future are:

_____

_____

_____

The areas for which I would like assistance and support to achieve my goals are:

_____

_____

_____

My action steps to get in the game and achieve those goals are:

_____

_____

_____

My list of specific goals and dates I wish to accomplish them include:

_____

_____

_____

Possible obstacles to watch out for (i.e., fear of rejection, fear of change, and lack of accountability, denial, lack of focus, lack of self-evaluation, lack of mentoring relationships):

_____

_____

_____

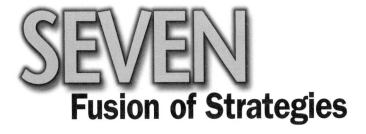

SEVEN
Fusion of Strategies

Those on the top of the mountain did not fall there. • **Unknown**

Patient Management 102
by Donna M. Sirvydas, R.D.H., M.Ed.

Since graduating from dental hygiene school, I have marveled at the biological, physiological, and technological ways in which dentistry continues to revolutionize itself. However, I am troubled, as well: Despite innovative strides made in disease prevention, restorative interventions, and effective oral-health education, there remains a recognizable barrier in the implementation of these services. The hurdle we dental professionals have yet to clear is the age-old challenge of successfully persuading patients to commit to the treatment plans we wholeheartedly present. Endless are the articles and seminars that aim to support our attempts at treatment planning and marketing. So why is it that we still struggle with the frustration of non-compliant patients?

One might—and many do—offer the view that the average layperson merely fails to understand and value the importance of his or her oral health; that dental treatment for most, takes its place below cars, vacations, medical treatment, and perhaps everything else on life's priority list. While this may be true, it's also true that cows will jump over the moon before a meticulous Power Point presentation, the promise of a Hollywood smile, or a consequential fear tactic changes all that. So, what will? I believe we need to bring the focus of our search for success with patient management back to the source: the patient.

It has been said that knowledge is power. If that's true, then the real key to success in dealing with dental patients lies in the knowledge of people—understanding human nature and the power of human relations. Okay, I know what you're thinking: The last thing you want to read about is a new-fashioned method to bring the "warm and fuzzies" to your patient care! Rest assured, this is *not* what I have in mind. Just as gimmicks don't work in dentistry, they don't work in human relations, either.

Successfully managing patients is similar to developing a skill in any other field: Its success depends on understanding and mastering certain basic principles. It has been proven that 60 percent to 90 percent of all failures in the world of business are due to failures in human relations. It is my experience that the art of genuinely relating to patients is one of the most overlooked and under-practiced skills—and yet, we as clinicians could use this skill to our advantage.

No matter how you look at it, we are in the "people" business, and whether you choose to evaluate success from purely a business-profit standpoint or a relational standpoint, one fact remains the same: There must be a two-way give and take. That means giving people what they want in return for what you want—a mutual exchange of benefits. Let's be honest: We want things from our patients—even *need* things from our patients—in order to enjoy successful practices. We want and need them to show up for their appointments, to pay their bills, to accept our treatment plans, and to follow through with those treatments without question or complaint. Not too much to ask, you might think. What do we give them in return—oral health? Perhaps; but arguably, we've already established that's not a priority for the majority of our patients. So, let me rephrase: What do our patients want (or more importantly, need) that we aren't currently giving them?

While the catch phrase "Show me the money!" is what movie viewers fondly remember most from the movie *Jerry McGuire*, in a believable way the movie illustrates the inevitable universal success that accompanies genuine human relations. As a high-powered sports agent in a competitive and cut-throat industry, Jerry McGuire has it all, until he suddenly discovers his scruples and goes out on a limb by writing a 25-page, touchy-feely mission statement. In his mission statement, entitled "The Things We Think, But Never Say: A Suggestion for the Future of our Company," he boldly shames the industry for chasing the almighty buck at all costs without forethought or genuine caring for the athletes they, as agents, represent. He further professes that the key to success lies in developing personal relationships—fewer patients, less money—and providing personal attention and caring. Soon after this epiphany, he loses his job, his fiancée, all but one of his clients, and struggles merely to survive, until he is forced to live up to his own mission statement. In doing so, the attention and caring he reluctantly prescribes to his professional and personal relations spawns a domino effect of success, happiness, and, of course, a landslide of "Show me the money."

While I'm not suggesting that dental practices reduce their patient population in order to provide a Zen of personalization, I am suggesting that we develop and maintain a concentrated focus on how we relate to our patients. As mentioned, in order to do this, we must first acquire a basic understanding of human nature.

Lesson #1: *All human behaviors are motivated by needs.* Throughout the years, many renowned theorists, psychologists, psychiatrists, counselors, motivational coaches, and the like have offered unique structures, values, perspectives, and relevance concerning how to better understand human nature and human behavior. Interestingly, despite their differences in personality and developmental theory, one central theme emerges: Human beings have an innate need and desire to feel important. That is: to feel that they are valued, appreciated, and significant.

Keep in mind that in order to successfully attain what we need from our patients, we must first give them what they need. In recognizing and acknowledging that our patients are motivated first and foremost by the desire to feel important, we can begin to effectively tap into the power of influence we possess.

We *all* possess the power to enhance our patients' feelings of personal worth. Making someone feel important, appreciated, and accepted is simple, if not necessarily easy. As our sense of personal worth is, to a large extent, based upon the reflections of the feelings that others have (or appear to have) about us, we need to be forever conscious of how our words and actions reflect to others. Therefore, the quickest way to improve human relations with your patients is to pay attention to the little things you say and do.

Have you ever recognized the fact that we notice only those things that are important to us? In any situation, we select for attention only those things that we consider necessary and important. In the process, we inadvertently miss valuable insights about what may be important to others. If we train ourselves to be present in the moment—to see, hear, and notice as much as we can about our patients—they will ultimately share with us all we need to know about them, thereby providing us with avenues by which we can persuade and influence them.

Let's first take a glance at your daily interactions and communications with your patients. Begin with how you receive patients from the waiting room or reception area in your office. Take note of how you meet and greet your patients, and remember that the first moment of contact will set the mood for the entire appointment, thus influencing your success at relating with them. Remind yourself of the fact that they need to feel important and notice them—really notice them! Make a lasting impression by giving them your undivided attention. Remember that your first words, actions, and attitudes invariably set the stage for your ability to succeed in managing that patient.

Don't underestimate the power of courtesy and politeness, and all those things that fall under the umbrella of what we refer to as manners. It is most often by the small courtesies that we acknowledge the importance of others. Make and keep eye contact while saying "Hello." Then, when you inevitability ask (as you should) that oh-so-routine question, "How are you today?" prepare yourself to listen (not merely hear), but truly *listen* to the response. Are you thinking, "Oh, I do that! I'm always attentive to my patients as I greet them."? Consider how many times you might pose this greeting in any given day. Do you actually *listen* to people's answers? Most of the time, you probably do not. Think back to yesterday's patients, or the last time you ran into an acquaintance at the grocery store. Can you remember what they said when you asked them, "How are you? How their day was going?" Again: We tend to notice only what is important to us. By genuinely noticing and paying attention to what people do and say, we are paying them a huge compliment, because we are reflecting back to them that we recognize their importance.

As we move past greetings to the clinical component of the dental appointment, we must continue to be conscious of how we notice, attend to, and relate to our patients—staying present in the moment, focusing on them and only them. Not just their dentition, but "them" as a person hungering for a sense of importance and acceptance. If you're anything like me, in a routine prophy appointment, you can update a patient's medical history, whip off an FMX, do a complete prophylaxis and a peri-odontal charting, while at the same time make a mental grocery shopping list, dream up your next family vacation, and map out your plan to fit in time to do laundry, supper, and pay the bills prior to sitting down to watch "Everybody Loves Raymond."

Recognizing that our human nature pays attention to only what is important to us, you can see how easy it is to be present everywhere but in the moment at hand—our patient's moment.

Despite the fact that our clinical tasks can lend themselves to minimal verbal communication with our patients, we would be wise to be especially attentive to what little they *do* have the opportunity to say. Remember that our power of influence depends upon our ability to fulfill our patients' need to feel important and accepted, and that that power is key to effective-ly persuade patients toward dental treatments—especially those who have resisted our efforts, time and time again. Once again, we must learn to work with human nature, instead of against it.

However, when we attempt to persuade another person to accept our viewpoint, ideas, or recommendations, we naturally tend to do just the opposite: The natural thing to do when we come up against a contrary idea, opinion, or a calculated excuse as to why the necessary dental treatment is not an option, is to argue our case. We debate. We pull out all the stops to cleverly convince our patients to accept what we have to say. Yet, the harder we try to force an idea, the more resistance that idea meets. We make ourselves out to be an opponent to our patients. We set up a verbal arena in which our patients find it necessary to defend themselves and their justifications. If we don't make them feel important and their viewpoints significant, they will make every effort to do it for themselves. Tell a person her ideas are stu-pid, and she will defend them all the more. Disregard a person's fears or ridicule his views and he will immediately close his mind to *your* ideas, no matter how valid they may be. We need to train ourselves to avoid this method of persuasion. It doesn't work!

What does work is the simple (not easy) art of listening and the subtle skill of suggestion.

The case of Mr. Jones

Consider Mr. Jones. He has resisted your recommendation for periodontal treatment for years. Upon arriving for his recare appointment, he undoubtedly knows you will once again try to convince him to succumb to treatment. He already has his mind closed to your attempts to persuade and has his artillery of defense arguments in order. So, round and round you go, each trying to convince the other to see things your own way.

You will succeed in stopping this merry-go-round and opening Mr. Jones' mind to your way of thinking to the degree that you succeed in acknowledging and accepting his.

Let him state his case—and listen to it. Don't interrupt and don't set the stage for a debate. Ignoring, interrupting, and brushing off what he has to say will only reflect that you view his thoughts, fears, concerns, and excuses as insignificant—and, thus, so is he. Until he has had the opportunity to say his piece and recognize that he was heard, he will not be open to what you have to say. As mentioned, our natural impulse when confronted with a viewpoint with which we don't agree is to argue; our minds are intuitively trained to immediately begin to mentally formulate our rebuttal. What happens next is communication suicide: We stop listening to the other person altogether. We are so busy getting ready to pounce and ram our own ideas down their throats the second they stop talking (or even before), that we don't listen to what they are actually saying.

That's why those skilled in the art of persuasion have mastered the art of listening. Give your undivided attention while listening. Show people that you are genuinely interested in their point of view by asking them to elaborate on their thoughts. Ask them questions relating to what they said. Then go one step further and repeat their thoughts back to them, so they know you truly listened—and heard.

Once Mr. Jones recognizes you have heard him, he will naturally let down some of the defenses he has built up. By listening, you have expressed to him that he is worth listening to and that you view him and his thoughts as important. You can now make him more willing to hear what *you* have to say by applying what psychologist Carl Rogers refers to as "unconditional positive regard." In your response to Mr. Jones, express that you empathetically understand and appreciate and even *agree* with what he has said. Remember, people love to think they're right and to feel their thoughts have value and merit. Resist the urge to argue and find fault in their views. In human relations, it doesn't always work to your advantage to prove yourself right 100 percent of the time. Skillful persuaders will always surrender some point of view in order to find a point of agreement. It is easier to persuade with a common focal point from which to start.

Listen carefully to be able to find that common focal point. Once you have completely and effectively listened to Mr. Jones' resistance, pause for a moment before you reply. This will once again let him know that you find what he has said as important—so much so that you are reviewing it and considering it. Then, while starting with your mutual point of agreement, state your case with low-pressure, subtly, again acknowledging his point of view. The goal here is not to replace his views with yours, but rather to slide yours in alongside. If he has already made a strong commitment to his defenses, the best you can do is skillfully plant a seed that will germinate later. State your case and let it go. Don't count on immediate results or attempt to force the issue, even if you recognize a glimpse of acceptance and conformity in his eyes. If you have managed to persuade him, allow him all the space and time he needs—even if it means six months from now—to tell you so on his own terms. If he agreed with you on the spot, after presenting a strong case against you, that would mean that he's admitting that he was wrong, and his need to feel important won't easily let him do that. Leave the door open for him to retreat and re-enter without sacrificing his ego. A successful persuader develops a talent for planting an idea, then wisely allowing the other person time to visualize the idea and present it later, as his or her own.

Successful patient management is all about getting patients to participate in our ideas. Keeping in mind that we need our patients—probably more than they think they need us—we must polish our people skills and work *with* the dynamics of human nature, rather than against them.

Developing and maintaining a concentration in human relations and effective communications mean much more than being a good conversationalist who has a repertoire of clever things to say. Only by careful listening and building awareness can we genuinely understand and accept others. And it is only through their acceptance of us that we have the power to influence *them*.

Communication: The Key to Success

by Bobbi Anthony, R.D.H.

As we have seen, no other skills in life can be more important to success than our ability to relate and communicate with each other. Our success as parents, spouses, employees, and leaders all require the establishment of quality relationships.

In his book, *Emotional Intelligence,* Daniel Goleman introduces the concept of emotional intelligence (EI) as something even more important than the Intelligence Quotient (IQ). He says, "How we handle ourselves and our relationships can determine life success, even more than IQ."

In a dental practice, almost everything that takes place depends on one kind of relationship or another. Whether it is the relationship between and among team members and patients, each other, or their employers, the ability to communicate effectively is one of the most important factors to success. Yet, the ability to communicate and create quality relationships is rarely taught as part of our general or higher educational process.

According to studies on job satisfaction, the emotions people experience while they're working reflect most directly the true quality of their work life. The percentage of time that people feel positive emotions at work turns out to be one of the strongest predictors of satisfaction and, therefore, of how likely employees are to stay or quit.

Quality relationships and effective communication require some of the same skills: the ability to listen with openness; to empathize; to relate; to be self-aware; to be fair and nonjudgmental; and the ability to cooperate.

In his book, *Primal Leadership,* Goleman and his partners take this concept even further.

The 'Group IQ'—the sum total of every person's best talents contributed at full force—depends upon the group's emotional intelligence, as shown in its harmony. A leader skilled in collaboration can keep cooperation high and thus ensure that the group's decisions will be worth the effort of meeting. Such leaders know how to balance the group's focus on the task at hand with its attention to the quality of members' relationships. They naturally create a friendly but effective climate that lifts everyone's spirits.

He goes on to say that those who spread "bad moods" are simply bad for business, while those who pass along "good moods" help drive a business's success. Since, for the most part, these skills of communicating and relating to each other are not taught in schools, church, or home; and if these skills could determine our life success, then isn't it important to create a strategy for mastering them?

Personality differences

Whether at work or home, teamwork and motivation are pivotal; so it seems reasonable that personality differences can actually help to determine success or failure. These personality differences can create joy and fun, or frustration and anger. They are what make life rich and fascinating, or frustrating and defeating. It is all in the way we see it.

One of the biggest awakenings in my life was when I finally realized that "I" make things mean what they mean. I accept people for their differences and diversities and use the shared knowledge of the group, or I take people wrong, based on the fact that I see issues differently than do they. This can cause me to refuse to deal with some people and to have as little to do with others as possible, simply because they don't see life or issues as I see them. I may express it by saying, "I don't like their personalities and I don't want them on my team," but in other words—they are just so different!

In their book, *The Platinum Rule,* Tony Alessandra, Ph.D., and Michael O'Connor, Ph.D., state that many people simply ricochet through life and never figure out why they can get along great with some people, yet cannot bear to deal with many others. They state that if more people understood the secret of "the differences among us," they would find that there is a very simple, but proven, way to build rapport with nearly everyone. They could then eliminate personality conflicts and take charge of their own compatibility with others. They could make business and personal relationships beneficial instead of a contest of wills. They call this the Platinum Rule.

The Golden Rule states, "Do unto others, as you would have them do unto you." The Platinum Rule bends the Golden Rule by stating that it is better to "Do unto others as they would have it done unto them." In other words: Learn how to really understand others, and then handle them in a way that is best for *them,* not just what's best for *us.* "It means taking the time to figure out the people around us," Alessandra and O'Connor say, "and then adjusting our behavior to make them more comfortable. It means using our knowledge and our tact to try to put others at ease."

Four hundred years before Christ was born, Hippocrates originated the idea that there are four basic "temperaments" or "personality styles." He described them with words not used as frequently today: phlegmatic, sanguine, melancholy, and choleric. In 1928, William Moulton Marston, Ph.D., published his work on behavioral styles in his book *Emotions of Normal People.* (Alessandra and O'Connor similarly offer an explanation for human behavior that is based on emotions.) Many of us have learned about his theories through more contemporary works based on his findings. The DiSC Personality Profiles distributed by Inscape Publishing are an example of current products based on the original concepts of Hippocrates and Marston.

I first experienced the DiSC Profiles in the early 1990s. The company (then called Carlson Learning) had developed personality surveys as instruments for learning more about ourselves—our strengths and our weaknesses. I was astounded when the survey outcome described me in incredible detail! I was so excited about sharing the knowledge that I have since become involved as a facilitator and distributor of the Inscape Products. I am constantly amazed at the measurements' reliability and the excitement displayed by many participants in my courses. It's as if I have new eyes by which to judge the world. I don't need to make others wrong based upon differences I have with them. I can accept their diversities and be thankful for their gifts—gifts that may not be my own. I have found strength in diversity.

The DiSC tools assist in understanding the meaning of events as they are experienced. The products are designed to be sensitive to the thoughts, feelings, and behaviors that particular situations evoke and to guide the respondents through the process of interpreting and applying what they have learned.

How better to understand others, than to first understand ourselves! For me, the experience was truly life changing. I now see the world through different eyes—eyes without blinders. Marston described an individual's emotional response to a situation as follows:

Dominance: *When the environment is perceived as unfavorable and the person feels more powerful than the environment, he or she experiences a Dominant response. This means the person is motivated to initiate action, respond quickly, take certain risks, and go straight to the point. She or he may be less preoccupied with examining alternatives, building consensus, or taking the time to win people over to a point of view.*

Influence: When the environment is perceived as favorable and the person feels more powerful than the environment, he or she experiences a desire to Influence. This means the person is likely to approach other people, volunteer to lead, solicit help, speak persuasively, and attract attention. He or she may be less preoccupied with planning and problem solving or ensuring that others have a chance to share attention.

Supportiveness: When the environment is perceived as favorable and the person feels less powerful than the environment, he or she experiences an opportunity to be Supportive. This means the person is motivated to contribute toward goals shared with others, assuming that what is good for someone else is good for him or her, too. The person may be less inclined to be the focus of attention and prefers a more equal distribution of effort and rewards.

Conscientiousness: When the environment is perceived as unfavorable and the person feels less powerful than the environment, he or she responds conscientiously. This means the person works within an area of personal discretion to ensure that standards are met and personal integrity is maintained, and he or she acts in ways that are comfortable for him or her. The person is less inclined to try to change the environment but may plan how to take advantage of change when it occurs.

The DISC theory of Dr. Marston has been used to explain human behavior in two ways. One approach views human behavior as a set of traits. Traits are implied when someone is described by words such as "she is a high D" or "You can tell I am a high I." In this application, the DiSC Dimensions are used to describe a person as consistently dominant, influencing, supportive, or conscientious in their behavior. (However, few if any people behave in the same way in all situations!)

Another way of thinking about DISC theory is to use it as Marston developed it—to explain people's emotional reactions to particular situations or events. These applications view human behaviors as a reflection of the mental/emotional state a person is experiencing at the time. Since environments are dynamic, a person's responses are expected to be dynamic; again, it is unlikely that anyone always responds the same in varied situations.

Let's take this a step further by using the personality styles as a means of identifying certain patients or team members.

Dominant/Driver/Director style

Traits:

Outgoing

Task-oriented

Thinks fast, talks fast

Cuts to the chase

Highly focused

Competitive

Results-oriented

Leader

Gets things done

May arrive 10 minutes early for an appointment, or 10 minutes late. Wants to leave early as they may have another appointment or a meeting

May stand over the appointment coordinator until they are seated in a treatment room

May be distrustful

Is interested in image of success, but doesn't necessarily care if others like them

Likes results, but doesn't necessarily care about feelings of others to obtain them

When communicating with a "D":

Show respect

Cut to the chase

Keep things moving quickly

Don't waste their time or talk down to them

With aesthetics, speak to them about image of success, not just about it looking pretty

Be on time

Be sincere, give facts, but without a lot of emotion

Be assertive

Be decisive

Influencer/ Socializer style
Traits:

Outgoing, persuasive

People-oriented

Fun loving

Optimistic

Life of the party

Talkative. This is the patient that not only tells you about their vacation, they bring photos

Likes to be noticed

Can be disorganized and may arrive late, but with lots of stories about what happened along the way

Can be disorganized or forgetful

Dislikes routine or loss of prestige

Cares if others like them

When communicating with an "I":

Show enthusiasm

Recognize them, never ignore them

Have fun with them

With aesthetics, tell them how great they will look

Be sincere and show your heart

Talk about feelings, not facts

Supportive/Steady/Relater style

Traits:

People-oriented

Likes one-on-one relationships versus public speaking

More introverted than extroverted

Easy going

Dislikes conflict

Servicing tendencies/likes to be helpful

Kind and a good listener

Accepting of others

Stable, good worker

Tends to hold feelings inside

Over-sensitive

Non-competitive

Can be indecisive

Dislikes insensitivity

When communicating with an "S":

Be patient/don't push

Listen

Let them move at their own pace

Don't confront or show anger

With aesthetics, allow them to be part of the solution

Give them time to adjust

Make them feel supported in a good relationship

Don't ignore their needs. As patients, they may not say they're upset—they just won't come back

Don't make too many sudden changes

Let them feel safe

Give reasons why the solution is in everyone's best interest

Be sensitive

Conscientiousness/Cautious/Thinker/Analytical style
Traits:

Reserved

Task-oriented

More introverted

Adheres to high standards

Wants to do the right thing

Not necessarily influenced by others

Likes accuracy and thoroughness

Analytical thinking

Talented and creative

Introspective

Deep and easily depressed

Possibly more socially insecure

May be a perfectionist and overly critical

Likes progress toward their goals

When communicating with a "C":

Don't criticize them or their work

Don't "make them wrong"

Be diplomatic

Stick to facts, not emotions

Let them help to find the solutions

Give them reasons why

Give them lots of details

With patients, talk about function and saving more of their natural tooth structure (not aesthetics)

Discuss health and doing the right thing for them

How to use this information

Many of the quality practices with which I have worked over the years have learned about personality styles and how to use this information to better communicate with team members and with patients. However, like anything we learn in life, repetition and study are necessary to make these techniques viable on a daily basis. If you and your team haven't yet learned about DiSC, I highly recommend you get started. There are many books and courses that you can explore individually or as a group. Not only will the information make you a better communicator in the practice, it will be a gift that can generate more love and understanding with your family as well.

Preceptorship versus Professionalism

by Maria Perno Goldie, R.D.H., M.S

As a past president of the American Dental Hygiene Association (ADHA) and a dental hygiene professional, I have some very strong convictions about education versus preceptorship.

To begin, I feel that, as dental hygiene professionals, advanced education is not only desirable, but also essential. I believe (as does ADHA) that we should have baccalaureate entry level into the profession. Why, you ask, when an associate degree and certificate assure that dental hygienists are capable of providing good patient care?

Yes they do, as I can attest; I was there at one point in my career. However, we will never be recognized as true professionals until we increase the body of knowledge in dental hygiene and increase our educational standards. The perception of our profession to fellow professionals is critical if we are to achieve autonomy. In addition, dental hygienists must be thoroughly prepared both intellectually and clinically to deal with older patients (as our population becomes grayer), infectious diseases, oral manifestations of oral conditions, and many other aspects of oral health as a critical part of total health. Whether we like it or not, we are a vital part of the interdisciplinary health-care delivery system. Critical thinking and communication skills are every bit as important as scaling and polishing—if not more so!

That said, I want to address level-accredited dental hygiene programs versus preceptor training, such as the Alabama Dental Hygiene Program (ADHP).

Most dental hygienists that are graduated from an accredited two-year program have the equivalent of a three- or four-year education. I feel these individuals should get credit for that education, articulated into a bachelor's degree program, and graduate with an appropriate educational degree. So, when I speak about baccalaureate entry level, I am not discounting the thousands of dental hygienists who do not hold a bachelor's degree. Nor do I believe that they deliver inferior care. I simply believe that they should get proper credit for their educational achievements from the very rigorous dental hygiene educational programs that they have endured.

As far as preceptor training, rules governing the ADHP program do not specify curricula or clinical competencies, as the programs accredited by the Commission on Dental Accreditation (CODA) specify. An analysis of the ADHP program shows that the ADHP program lacked the following courses specified by CODA, in course hours:

- Period ontology (42 hours)
- Nutrition (28 hours)
- Head and neck anatomy (33 hours)
- Pathology (10 hours)
- Public health (40 hours)
- Dental materials (42 hours)
- Law and ethics (20 hours)
- English (88 Hours)

- Speech, psychology (44 hours)

- Sociology (44 hours)

- Chemistry (144 hours)

- Pharmacology (48 hours)

- Oral embryology and histology (22 hours)

The biggest problem I have with the faculty of the ADHP is educational methodology. That is: Faculty in CODA-accredited programs must be well qualified in specific curricular subject matter, current dental-hygiene functions, and educational methodology; they must be part of a core of qualified, full-time faculty and evaluated by a formal, objective system of faculty evaluation. In the ADHP program, any dentist who is licensed and practicing dentistry in Alabama, full-time, can be a trainer.

However, there is no mandate that they be qualified in educational methodology—so how do they know how to teach? They have no formal dental hygiene education—so what do they know about dental hygiene? There is no specification concerning a current library, facilities such as a laboratory, classroom space, offices for administration, or radiographic facilities. Instructional aids and resources are not specified, either. And, to make matters worse, all of this training takes place in the dentist's for-profit dental office!

"Meeting in the middle" is not an acceptable method of negotiation when a patient's health and public safety are at stake. Dental hygienists are still required to work under the direct supervision of a dentist in Alabama, which is contradictory to cost-effective delivery of dental hygiene services. It is also contradictory to being a professional, if you view the characteristics of a profession.

Does this situation exist because educational requirements are minimal or because dentists want to exercise control? *General* supervision is in effect in many states and other countries around the world, and it enables well-educated dental hygienists to safely and effectively render their services in a cost-efficient manner.

As licensed health-care providers, we are responsible for the care we render and for the safety of the patient. While I believe that dental-hygiene professionals should work collaboratively with other professions (including dentistry), I do not view that role as ancillary to dentistry or a vocation that supports dentistry. Dental hygiene is a profession unto itself. We must persevere to achieve autonomy, build our body of knowledge, increase membership in our professional association, and achieve all of the characteristics that make us responsible professionals.

Our venue may be a dental office, our own office, a hospital, a public-health setting, or any other number of settings, but we are ultimately responsible for the care we render. It may be as an employee, an employer, an independent contractor, a business owner, an educator, a researcher, an administrator, a sales person, a consultant, or any number of roles of which we are capable. Formal education is a vital part of the preparatory process for any of the roles dental hygiene professionals undertake.

Choose Wisely: Design Your Focus

Employment benefits and perks: Things to consider, negotiate, plan, and write out

Full/Part time

Are duties and responsibilities defined?

Written job description?

Working hours:

Work days:

Lunch period:

When working hours vary, you will be notified in the following manner:

Salary

Starting rate: $ per

Gross salary:

Commission (%):

Paid vacations? With full salary?

Paid holidays?

Paid sick leave/"well" pay?

Bonus paid?

Continuing education and travel benefits?

Uniforms?

Professional association membership?

Pension and/or profit sharing?

What is the vesting schedule?

Who is vested?

Disability insurance provided?

Life insurance provided?

Medical or dental care provided?

Malpractice (separate policy than owner) insurance provided?

Practice-sponsored dental services: Team members, who have access to practice-sponsored dental services. Team members should include the value of those services in your compensation mindset, and own your own problem/desires, etc. just like patients must own theirs. Team members must participate actively in making choices for themselves.

Eligibility for benefits:

There may be specific waiting periods before certain things kick in, depending on the office

Official office manual?

Conditions of employment:

What is the review process?

First Review In   Days

Second Review In   Days

Third Review In   Days

Reviews Thereafter:

Conditions for Termination:

Team careers and professions—not just jobs

Are there quality people for whom you choose to build something great?

- Join professional associations that support your knowledge curriculum, (ADHA, ADAA, ADA, AACD, ADIA, and PM)

- Hang your diploma, certification, and license on the wall

- When treating teachers/educators, offer the opportunity for you to come speak to their classes and/or receive information for a unit on oral health.

- Contact, and make yourself available, to the local newspaper's health editor. Volunteer to be called every time an article about oral health is planned.

- Add your name to the list for career days in the area schools

- Stay connected!

- Go to association-sponsored events and meet the officers/members

- Continually educate patients on what you do and what schooling is required to get licensed.

- Be a professional (look at what you do as a career, not as something you do until lunch)

Do you know . . .

. . . what type of supervision your area requires for hygienists for the following functions and duties?

If you are unsure, contact your state dental or dental hygiene committee/board. And if you are legally allowed to perform some functions for which you are not yet qualified, ask yourself—why aren't I qualified?

- Hygiene diagnosis—assessment/examination

- Intra- and extra-oral examinations

- Periodontal and restorative charting
- Local anesthesia
- Nitrous oxide analgesia
- Root planing
- Laser periodontal therapy
- Curettage
- Local antimicrobial therapy
- Subgingival irrigation
- Microbiological analysis
- Place and remove periodontal dressings
- In-office whitening
- Laser whitening
- Pit and fissure sealants
- Restorative polishing and renewing
- Restorative placement, contour, and polymerization
- Other functions not listed above

Do you know . . .

. . . what type of supervision and expanded-function require-ments your area requires for certified dental assistants for the fol-lowing duties?

If you are unsure, contact your state dental or dental assisting committee/board. And if you are legally allowed to perform some functions for which you are not yet qualified, ask yourself: Why aren't I qualified?

- Pit and fissure sealants
- X-rays
- Fluoride
- Topical agents

- Coronal polish
- Remove supragingival cements/deposits
- Chart existing restorations
- Take impressions
- Fabrication of nightgaurds
- Fabrication of whitening trays
- Fabrication of provisionals
- Placement of provisionals
- Whitening therapy
- Orthodontic services

And on the flip side: If you are a team member who is performing functions without the proper license or expanded function qualifications, then get them! Take pride in yourself and in your abilities. Do not allow anyone to compromise your ethical excellence or patient care.

Is insurance good for hygiene? Well, maybe . . .

If a team member considers the influence that insurance plays in dental and hygiene care, then he or she may begin to understand that many dental insurance plans are *not* structured to promote oral health or allow you to achieve financial gain.

Sleeping with the enemy

Many registered dental hygienists are working with liaison groups to help promote an autonomous dental hygiene profession. But choose your bedfellows wisely!

In our pursuit to be recognized as a care provider who can be reimbursed directly for hygiene services, we need to learn from the many dental mistakes. If, in your area, you can bill and get direct reimbursement for hygiene services, can you only charge the patient the set insurance companies' "reasonable and customary" fees? Once you have calculated your overhead and established the desired hourly salary you want to receive, the insurance payment may leave you short. In some instances—in an effort just to break even—it may cause you to provide superficial hygiene services—the very situation we often complain about when working for doctors/employers.

Blindly aligning yourself with an HMO or an insurance company may seem proactive at first, but in the long run you may just be swapping signatures on your paycheck (from employee-dentist to employee-insurance company) without achieving any real autonomy!

Lastly, if your current employment situation has a strong insurance dependence, that may be why you are asked to treat 25 patients in one day and haven't gotten a raise in two years. Determine your hourly overhead with full employment salary package, and then subtract the fee assigned to the services you provide. You may be surprised to discover how much or how little is left over. Remember: One fundamental goal of any business is to take in more money than it pays out.

Distinction

The entire team is responsible for the distinctive services and the impact that the office makes on your patients. How well the team does this will influence patient retention and referrals.

Team action meeting

- Establish regular team meetings
- Assign a rotating facilitator
- Assign an action plan coordinator
- Establish agenda items
- What is currently working or not working within your office that supports or does not support the vision?
- Schedule a time allotted during the team meeting for each idea
- Assign a team member to take responsibility for specific agenda items

- Establish a target date for the action idea implementation and feedback circle/ meeting

Cancellation strategy

A patient calls to cancel or break an appointment—or just outright misses one. This leaves an opening in the schedule. What system is in place to fill the opening?

Most missed-appointment systems do nothing more than attempt to bring in an already-scheduled patient earlier. The problem? This adds virtually no production to the schedule!

How do *you* track no-shows and cancellations? Do you use some form of a computerized management system? Do you call patients who miss or do you wait for them to call the office? Are you even able to identify habitual offenders when they make appointments, or do you just put them into the schedule without auditing their chart and past appointment patterns?

Can you even audit this type of information? Do you have an office procedure with which to check? Is it a part of your office protocol to proactively follow up with appointment offenders? How effective are you in this effort?

Many teams are missing an opportunity to add production, retrain patients on their appointment policies, and maintain a more loyal patient base.

Distinctive patient education: A checklist

- CAESY/Smile Channel available in the offices.
- Create one-page information sheets that offer patient education on oral hygiene or post-operative care. This helps to ensure that patients leave your office feeling educated and with an appreciation for the value received in your care. This can also be done via e-mail.
- Use models, books, illustrations, and digital imaging to educate patients.
- If patients view videos or computer programs in private about conditions and/or treatments, offer each patient a clipboard with paper and pencil to write down questions.

- Have a photo album of your own work in your guest area and hygiene room. Be sure to have the album labeled and have it easily accessible to patients. Include captions that explain the patient's story as well as the condition and the treatment.

Dental and hygiene spas

- Offer patients comforts in the guest area, like healthy beverages, muffins, or fruit.
- Aromatherapy units can aid in pleasantly freshening office air and soothing patients.
- Purifiers may clean the air of odors.
- Warm towels may help patients feel refreshed and pampered after treatment.
- *Shiatsu* neck massagers are wonderful for patient relaxation between steps of long procedures. Or, hire a massage therapist to visit the office during long-treatment sessions.
- Provide headset-tape players or radios that patients control
- Place fresh flowers at the front desk.
- Offer a phone line in your reception area for patient use or use as a modem hook-up.
- Greet and acknowledge patients personally.
- Rethink the "before" pictures in reception or treatment areas. Patients may find them distasteful. When was the last time you visited a hair salon and viewed bad hair day photos on the wall?

Survival skills: Finding the weakest link

What is the weakest link in your office? Finding the weak links in your office is key to gaining and retaining patients and earning patient referrals. Objectively review the following questions and evaluate those areas where there are weaknesses.

- Discuss congruence in your public image.
- How well do your office location, building appearance, and collateral materials (such as phone communications) "speak" about you? Are you congruent in these areas?

- When you send out materials to new patients, do they accurately represent who you are?
- From the moment the patient enters your door until he/she departs the office, how well do you maintain consistency in the quality of service? Are you congruent and consistent?
- For your patients of record, are you consistent from appointment to appointment?
- How are you getting feedback from your patients? (*Are* you getting feedback from your patients?)
- Do you conduct surveys; hold focus groups; have a consistent level of quality that you establish early in the relationship with the patient?
- Do you conduct patient advisory groups?
- What can you do to ensure you have your fingers on the pulse of your patients?

Receptionist/Appointment Administrator/Treatment Coordinator: Will you . . .

- Speak confidently about the office, doctor, and hygienists when patients call? (Please stop saying, "Oh the girl will be able to clean your teeth this week." Use team members' names when talking to patients.)
- Greet patients warmly when they arrive at the office?
- Shake hands, say hello, and introduce yourself, using first and last names? Perhaps wear a name badge?
- Thank them for choosing your practice?
- Use formal salutations until otherwise directed by the patient?
- Verbalize patient value if appropriate to the appointment?
- Build rapport with the patients?
- Pass patients off to the clinical team for safekeeping until treatment?
- Further discuss the recommendations the clinical team is making and help them understand the conditions of their mouth?
- Handle scheduling and financial arrangements?

• Track the progress of the case and make sure of appointments?

Lunchtime whitening or lunchtime peel

The dental office atmosphere can be private and relaxing if you add amenities like massage chairs and consider the personal music selection—so why not look into added-value services?

One such service deals with power whitening and another with microdermabrasion. In many cases, both procedures can be delivered by a trained team member under minimal or no doctor supervision in the interest of improving your patient's appearance.

No longer a B2

If your team is committed to aesthetics, but still only recording a shade B2 on a majority of lab slips, determine why. Natural teeth are not monochromatic, so why would laboratory-processed or single-visit (CEREC restorations) be? Learn the skill of staining/glazing or detailed shade selection and recording. (Figs. 7–1, 7–2, 7–3).

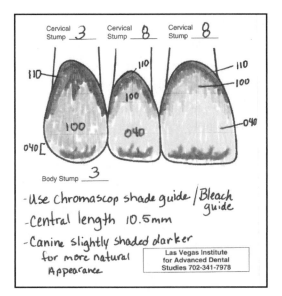

Fig. 7–1: *Example of an anterior color map, courtesy of the Las Vegas Institute of Advanced Dental Studies.*

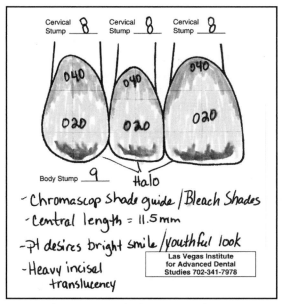

Fig. 7–2: *Example of an anterior color map,*
courtesy of the Las Vegas Institute of Advanced Dental Studies.

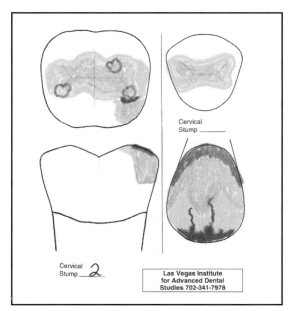

Fig. 7–3: *Example of a posterior color map,*
courtesy of the Las Vegas Institute of Advanced Dental Studies.

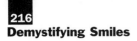

Fresh breath strategy

Update yourself on the connection between volatile sulfur compounds and gingivitis and periodontal disease. The newest therapeutic information may sway nay-sayers to look or look again at clinical rationales for stocking appropriate self-care systems in their offices for their patient's oral and systemic health.

Quoting fee strategy

Stay off the slippery slope of itemizing every fee for every service during discussions with patients. At one time or another, a patient will challenge fees, question whether they really need the doctor's exam today, or say "Hold off on those x-rays until next time!"

Instead, quote a complete fee for a hygiene or restorative procedure. For example, "It will be $300 for your hygiene visit!"

Websites: Do you shine?

By now, a large percentage of practices drawn to this book have a presence on the Internet. What I would like team members to evaluate is your inclusion in it.

Does it have a team section?? Does it include a photo and biographical sketch of each member? If not— why not?

Get your head in the game

- To whom does your office refer for periodontal therapy, orthodontics, and/or oral surgery?

- Do you know what the month-to-date gross goal and collection goal is?

- Who are your new patients today?

- Are there open hygiene or doctor times today?

- Have you reviewed your patient's charts for unscheduled or unfinished periodontal or restorative treatment?

- Do your patients have complete periodontal charts, intra-oral pictures, up-to-date necessary radiographs, etc.?

- Are your radiographs out on the view box or on the computer monitor during appointments?
- Do you perform oral cancer examinations on all patients?
- Have you made any post-session phone calls?
- Do you believe in yourself?
- Will you take a chance to move yourself and your profession?

Communication strategy: When you treat your patients, do you . . .

- Take the time to learn what is important to them?
- Set aside your agenda so you can learn theirs?
- Involve them in the decision-making?
- Ask them to participate in their care?
- Support them as they struggle with limitations of time, money, energy, and other issues?

Sample smile dialog

A clinician does not have to sound robotic or memorize scripts in order to discuss smile enhancement options with patients. Quite the opposite. You can be direct and clear, but shift your focus from *telling* to *asking* and bring graciousness to your patient's discussions. Get curious about what the patient is thinking.

"Mrs. Jones, I've noticed that two of your front teeth are darker than the others. Is that something you are aware of? Is it a concern to you?" Then: "I'd welcome the opportunity to help you change that. We have so many wonderful options available, and I wouldn't want to fall short of inviting you to consider them."

Establishing a communication protocol and team pre-evaluation of patient smiles can enhance summary discussions between the doctor and the team member.

Criteria for temporaries

Provisionals should mimic the natural tooth. The tooth/ teeth should have proper:

- Periodontal health
- Size
- Contour
- Shade
- Emergence profile
- Contacts
- Embrasures
- Occlusion
- Marginal fit

Why professionalism? Why now?

Why wouldn't a team member want to develop his/her professionalism, then manage and profit by it? Unfortunately, when asking members of the dental community what the term "professionalism" means or how it can benefit them and their delivery of quality care, the response is that they haven't a clue.

Nonetheless, professionalism and its management are untapped tools in a robust career lexicon. Team players have buried their heads in the sand far too long and relinquished to someone else accountability for the success or failure of their careers, their departments, and their practices.

Let's review some of the broad trends in dentistry and dental hygiene that seem to be significantly influencing the knowledge-sharing evolution:

- The competition in our industry
- The emergence of new practice ownership arrangements
- Dental management companies
- Employers cutting back on oral health benefits

These focuses put terrific pressure on dental offices and our professions for increased adaptability, flexibility, and service-intense practices. One of the best ways to respond to that pressure is to develop an awareness of the value of specialized knowledge—aesthetic dentistry, periodontology, implantlogy, etc.—as embedded in practice processes, routines, or teams.

Happily, the shift by dental and dental hygiene professionals away from performing drill and fill services, and wanting to perform more preventive, tooth preservation, and natural- appearing definitive treatments, is pacing the public's desire to shift from get-me-out-of-pain services to procedures that result in better oral health and more beautiful smiles. This mutual paradigm shift can be summarized this way:

- Awareness of the shift in focus to center or co-diagnosis dental offices

- Awareness of the increase in oral health-related, quality-of-life services

- More complete involvement of dental manufacturers in material science development

- Advances in technology relating to more efficient assessment, tracking, diagnostic, and communication tools

- Emerging and continual discussions supporting evidence-based practicing

We can argue for or against these trends; however, business industry leaders are discovering that businesses no longer just sell services and products, they are selling *knowledge*. Even in the dental industry, we are in the business of knowledge. This knowledge-intense business landscape also results from a trend toward "mass customization" (PPOs, HMOs, and DSP-media campaigning from dental manufacturers). As reflected in commercials, organized public service announcements, and other outlets, this trend is essentially building towards a greater knowledge of oral-health issues out of what used to be a relatively unknown service. However, in doing so, it does create distinctions.

For example: Many production-line dental offices schedule a cleaning every 30 to 45 minutes. More knowledge-intense, service-oriented offices schedule a non-surgical periodontal appointment or an oral-health appointment every 60 to 90 minutes. By checking around, people are discovering different levels of service. And the office that is able to translate a dental hygienist's knowledge base and value (in the above example) is better able to tailor services and stands to increase hygiene services with every visit, as well as increase referrals.

In what might otherwise be considered a commodity—dental cleanings—an office may see its profit margin widen by capitalizing on this knowledge and skill component.

In addition to a change in business thinking, knowledge management is also made necessary by the changing structure of dental practices—particularly the desire to integrate non-traditional services. Dental practices and their professional staffs, once organized along functions or titles (hygienist, chairside assistant, or office manager), are now reorienting themselves toward expanded roles, technologies, non-segregated total treatment plans, and individual passions of continual learning.

To better understand this change in thinking, let's look at "assets." Assets can be defined as everything a company owns that has value. Assets can be categorized into two groups: One group, precise and measurable, and one group with no physical existence. These groups make up tangible and intangible assets.

Established accounting mechanisms for business have evolved around companies' tangible assets. Examples of tangible assets are the facility, the equipment, fixed costs, and inventories. These assets show up on accounting statements as part of the book value of a practice. However, a company's value in the world market can range from two to 10 times the book value. This means the market values the company in excess of its tangible assets. This tells a simple, but profound truth: The hard assets of a company contribute far less to the ultimate value or worth of its service (or product) than the intangible assets.

Intangible assets are also termed "professional assets." Professional assets make up the difference between an accounting balance sheet and the actual value of the practice. A broad range of examples of dental/team members knowledge assets may include the employees' and doctor's knowledge (depth and breadth of their experience, talent, or expertise); patient satisfaction; service innovation; morale; patient preferences; relationships with patients; relationships with other health care professionals; the health of employer/employees, the employees' willingness to learn; how they apply information; clinical techniques and technologies; reputation; image; logo—anything and everything that may create the practice's competitive advantage!

There is a growing recognition and acceptance of knowledge as a measurable asset alongside assets such as land, labor, and capital that can be considered a greater force than any of the others in the production of services. Practices have long managed, analyzed, and reassessed land, labor, and capital; by contrast, we have only started to understand and analyze the workings of knowledge in dental offices.

Management visionary Peter Drucker coined the terms "knowledge worker" and "knowledge work" around 1960. My research reveals that in dentistry, Avrom E. King refers to the concept of "intellectual management practices" for dentistry in the late 1980s. Knowledge—the creation and management thereof—has been profiled as the primary business opportunity of the 20th century. Knowledge is now *the* commodity of business—not just *a* commodity of business.

The evolution of professional knowledge

The origin of knowledge capital (intellectual capital) dates to 1768, when a Swedish businessman pondered why his competition was twice as busy as he. He concluded that he used the same quality of materials as his competitors, but found "that it wasn't fixed assets (material)" that gave his competitors the upper hand but the "intelligence with which the machines were employed."

The change to a professional knowledge environment is directly influenced by the increase in the "value content" of a business' various jobs. In a dental practice, for instance, receptionists are no longer just people who turn pages of the appointment book and pencil in times and procedures. A majority of them no longer manually write out insurance forms or keep accounting books in longhand. These "administrators" utilize paperless communication; computer-generated insurance forms; faxes; e-mail; and computerized appointment schedules and accounting programs. They run and analyze reports rather than keeping a spiral notebook full of scratched out information; they no longer retype referral letters (using word processing software instead), and are perhaps even arranging continuing education sessions between referring offices.

Thanks to the information and technology explosion—and how practices have responded to it—patients no longer find stereotypical front desk receptionists, but professional workers with knowledge assets.

Knowledge assets, like other intangible professional assets, may not be very popular within our professions. As clinicians, we come from a scientific, research-based education. This concept of knowledge may feel abstract, fuzzy, or non-scientific. But we are beginning to realize that a skilled clinician may file bankruptcy while an average or below-average clinician may have to turn away referrals. Why the disparity? *"It's the people, stupid!"* We are determining that dentistry and dental hygiene are far more than skill-based professions. It's people-based— whether we mean the clinician, patient, repair specialist, laboratory technician, or sales person. Despite our unfamiliarity with the topic, knowledge *happens*!

For a moment, let's examine how our patients' knowledge is changing, how they are becoming informed about their health-care choices, and what they want or do not want.

Historically, patients seeking treatment were primarily pain-driven. As the benefits of fluoride became proven for use in prevention and the use of amalgam became popular as a restorative material, patients visited dental offices for treatment beyond crisis care. Now, consumers are learning about, and desiring, more healthy and sparkling smiles.

On the practitioner side, traditional dentists and hygienists have always been teeth-centered. Many professionals have tunnel vision, seeing only the tooth and soft tissue and wearing blinders when it comes to the patient's overall health and well-being. We have also been guilty of mounting our soapboxes to lecture to our patients about what they need or should do for their teeth, based on one-way communication. The result has been non-participatory involvement from the patient and limited behavioral change to support a healthy oral environment.

There are bountiful stories, however, that our professions are breaking out of their traditional characterizations and segregated treatment plans/services. Dentists are breaking away from the "Little Shop of Horrors" image to become smile artists or designers and providing quality-of-life services and/or "smile lifts." Dental hygienists have been mastering their positions and the language they use to describe the services they provide. They are changing the stereotype of "cleaning lady" to "oral-health educator or coach," prevention specialist, and/or patient health facilitator. Changing technology, demographics, education systems, value systems, political systems, social systems, and economics all influence these developments.

Oral health services must begin with "wholeness"—a health-centered practice embodying the alignment of oral fitness, overall health, and beauty. No longer will it be acceptable to have a hygiene treatment plan on the blue sheet and a restorative treatment plan on a yellow sheet. These services must be integrated and presented as complete care plans. These shifts partner dentistry with dental hygiene and with other aspects of the health and medical fields. They are no longer to be seen as separate entities; they are providing the foundation for knowledge-managed oral care. Knowledge is the link to providing value and quality care.

The many areas of professionalism can be clustered. One such cluster is *tacit knowledge* and the other is *explicit knowledge*. Tacit knowledge is the personal knowledge a person holds. It involves a person's experiences, education, values, purpose, perceptions, etc. Explicit knowledge is knowledge that can be codified or transferred to one person or another through systematic means. The significance here is that knowledge is interactive, moving from tacit to explicit all day long. The process of knowledge sharing can be further categorized into processes like socialization, internalization, externalization, and combinations within the clusters of tacit and explicit knowledge.

For example: During a morning huddle, when the office team is reviewing patient charts and discussing the day's schedule, knowledge sharing combines socialization and internalization. *Socialization* is the sharing of knowledge between people, tacit to tacit. *Internalization* is the transferring of knowledge from explicit to tacit—moving information from the chart or schedule to the practitioners. Once the practitioner has this explicit knowledge, he or she can use it to deliver services based on their own tacit assets.

An example of an externalization/tacit-to-explicit knowledge transfer comes when a dental hygienist inputs treatment notes into a computer or chart. A computer running a scan report or processing electronic insurance forms is a combination knowledge transfer—explicit knowledge to explicit knowledge. The terms are not important; what needs to be emphasized is how knowledge moves within our practices. We can develop patterns of learning and integrating knowledge into databases, processes, systems, or performance that can be directed, created, measured, and managed.

Professionals are human, too!

Dental practices can no longer afford to keep tacit knowledge (knowledge contained only within individuals' minds) in the gray matter of its employees, ceramists, or sales representatives. Employee knowledge and the management of that knowledge are what determines a dental office's differentiated advantage. The human side of professional assets can be described as a team member's knowledge, flavored by the individual's experiences, personal beliefs, perspectives, value systems, judgments, care, and specialized skills. Specialized skills that one brings to a job may include formal education, license, certifications, expanded work portfolio, bilingual abilities, sign language, a passion for holistic medicine, or mastery of a computer program. These attributes—which belong to the employee, but are used by the practice in return for salary and benefits—are part of the added value of the office.

An example of consciously hiring professionals occurred when my dental office interviewed for a dental hygiene position. Management had determined that its hygiene recare system had to be assessed for two additional clinical days per week. The practice had been moving in the direction of understanding behavioral aspects of providing care and co-discovering patient needs and desires. During the interviewing process, we were fortunate to speak with a hygienist who had broader expertise in facilitation and communication. The human capital she offered was the ability to provide clinical skills required of a hygienist while bringing to the game—and, ultimately, to the patients—a different, value-added skill, *i.e.,* facilitator.

Another example is the dental assistant preparing the armamentarium for a crown and bridge procedure. All things being equal, it appears to be a routine preparation. He gathers the needed instruments—always checking the office's detailed procedure manual, step-by-step outline, and/or treatment instrument picture guide. However, complications arise; the tooth is more structurally damaged than first expected. He calls upon his past experiences, thought processes, and decision-making abilities to anticipate additional needs the dentist and the patient have in order to successfully complete the procedure. This is not a matter of the dentist micromanaging the situation. The needed information in this case is not written in the procedure manuals. It is hard to foresee every obstacle, such as this one, but the assistant's past experiences add value to the office and the patients he serves.

(In this hypothetical situation, an assistant working in a knowledge-based dental office would schedule non-patient time to document this circumstance and end result. This analysis would then be incorporated into the general database for future retrieval when needed. Procedure manuals should not be dusted off every few months, but should be working documents, sometimes changing daily or hourly.)

A final example involves a business assistant working with patients. He eliminates possible embarrassing moments by quickly changing last names in the computer when patients divorce. He knows Mrs. Jones only wants to come in on Thursdays, Mr. Ends needs an early-morning appointment, and Mr. Long likes milk in his coffee when he is waiting for his wife. He establishes personal relationships with many of the claim officers at the insurance companies to which a majority of the patients subscribe—relationships that have helped speed up pre-authorization procedures or the release of reimbursement checks. He knows all of the sales people by name and often negotiates below-average pricing on supplies.

These are all examples of humans at work. The business assistant's knowledge is value-added for the patients.

(This hypothetical example of a team member's knowledge (tacit) can be transformed into a system of retrievable data (explicit) and, therefore, becomes a permanent practice resource (intellectual capital) of the office in the event the business assistant decides to leave his position. How many management systems provide areas for individualized notes that can detail the details? And, more important, how many practice atmospheres encourage team members to take the time to record such knowledge?)

Practices hire a variety of employees with a variety of competencies. Not all employees fall under the category of "professional." There is a difference between basic skills and professional skills. The basic skills of employees include reading and writing, or fundamental competencies needed to perform a job. An office should employ professional workers and the supporters of those workers as parts of the same team.

When discussing professional or team talents and skills, do not go into your offices and outwardly label who is and who is not a knowledge worker, or who is on the A team and who is on the B team. Nor should some members be thought of as superior and other workers made to feel somehow inferior. Employee development investing needs to evolve after the knowledge base of a practice has been analyzed.

During discussions with employers within the dental community, I often hear sentiments like, "Why should I invest money in her continued education, when I am not sure if she will be with me next year?" This thinking perpetrates the notion that an employee is a costly expense or a charitable contribution, rather than a valuable source of current and future wealth.

Here's an alternative way of thinking and practicing: What if all dental employers felt self-development contracts and continual learning was the norm, and their employees were given unlimited opportunities for growth? What if dentists invested in all team members? If a new hire came from an office that similarly invested in their team, wouldn't she also be a knowledge worker? What's more, if the office managed its knowledge effectively, then the tacit knowledge of all departing employees would be stored in a database, to be retrieved and used again and again, even after the person had moved on to another office.

Considering current business thinking, employers who do not see the need to continually create learning opportunities within their offices will no longer be in business. The business climate and competition will eliminate them.

It has also been my challenge to the professional to invest in *self*, creating ongoing expanded work and experience portfolios (provisional crown and bridge sealant placement, restoration renewal services, smile assessments, non-surgical laser therapy, administering local anesthesia, etc.), whether a current employer funds the learning or not. One needs to be loyal to his or her chosen professional discipline, and a team professional who grows will continue to ensure himself or herself a place as a knowledge worker. One who does not make the commitment voluntarily will find himself or herself involuntarily turned into a "spit-sucker, prophy king, or appointment juggler." Professionals without continual challenges (expanded functions) will find themselves the support or basic-skilled employees, due to the changing dental service economy.

Structural capital

Structural capital is the second category of intellectual capital. It can be defined as everything that remains when the people go home.

Research and development have opened doors to advances in structural capital in dental practices. The technological explosion aids in the assessment and prognosis of the patient, while improving the quality of care provided in a more cost-efficient manner. New technologies and applications in dentistry and dental hygiene include:

- Diagnostic instrumentation (caries detection, periodontal identification)
- Computerization (clinically and administratively)
- Intra-oral cameras/video
- Micro-dentistry (air abrasion)
- Digital radiography/cameras/imaging
- Lasers
- Advances in material science and techniques
- Advances in chemotherapeutics and localized periodontal therapies
- Intranet/Internet
- Tissue engineering
- Ultrasonics; mini-ultrasonics
- Advances in self-care products and solutions
- Gene therapy/microbiological testing

Computer use alone, as one part of structural capital in dentistry and dental hygiene, is used in areas of practice management, clinical work, continuing education, and patient communication. Computer applications in knowledge-practice management means decentralizing work centers and spreading the workload efficiently and effectively among the employees. One popular way this is done is by placing a network terminal in each operatory or at central locations throughout the office to allow communication among employees while preventing duplication of efforts.

To illustrate: In an office with limited computerization, the care provider makes documentation of the care provided, fills out the service-rendered information, the next-needed appointment, etc., in patients' records. They then give the chart to a person at the front desk, who most often verbally reiterates everything that was documented in the chart so the person at the front desk can appear to know what is going on with the patient's care. The front desk person then inputs this information into the computer in order to print out a bill or schedule another appointment. All of this happens while the patient is waiting! If a computer was located where each clinician could easily access it, and a system was set up to service a chartless office, all information could be entered chairside and the patient could leave with a printed bill, appointment card, or referral letter—and a better perception of value!

Computers can aid in efficiency with electronic billings, electronic treatment notes, transferring files, online scheduling, tracking personal information, insurance information, e-mail appointment confirmations, financial planning for the office and patients, processing forms, accounting, and referral letters to specialists. In addition, all of these functions can be completed with computers located either in the office or networked offsite.

Applications for clinical use include operatory-based computers for automated and voice-active charting, intra-oral cameras, digitized radiographs and photographs, medical and dental history updates, smile-design protocols, and documentation. In addition, the intra-oral camera with image, document, and storage-capture capabilities offers a form of visualization and communication previously unavailable to dentistry and dental hygiene. Imaging permits the capture, storage, retrieval, and presentation of visual information that can be transformed into knowledge for the team and education channels for the patient.

Radiographic and photographic images can be captured as digital information. Digital radiography—or reduced radiation exposure radiography—allows an image to be manipulated, rotated, magnified, and modified. Captured images can then be displayed electronically and used in treatment assessment, patient education, professional education, and documentation for correct diagnostic capabilities. Subtraction radiography allows assessment of an area by comparing two films through digital means.

CAD/CAM (computer-aided design and computer-aided manufacturing) can be applied to the fabrication of dental restorations. Information for the fabrication of dental restorations may come from scanning casts, dies, or from a computer-generated image of the prepared tooth as digital impressions.

All of these areas compement the human side of a dental practice while strengthening value for the patient.

The Internet is having a dramatic impact on dentistry and dental hygiene. Statistically, many people hate to go to the dentist; many feel at a disadvantage because they are apprehensive and not informed. A lot of patients are justifiably nervous, because they are not in control. This is an area where a well-designed web site can benefit the patient. Dental offices can take this opportunity to transform themselves and add real value for the patient by becoming information-rich health centers. People will still need to go into a dental office to get provided services, but they do so as better-informed consumers. Prior to picking up the phone or e-mailing for an appointment, a patient can determine from a well-developed web site:

- Where the dentist received training/biographical information/training

- How long he or she has been in practice

- Location of the dental office, the educational levels of the dental team, billing policies, infection control/ patient protection policies, hours of operation, and office philosophy

- Who the dentist refers to (why and for what), as well as review a copy of the office newsletter and letters from satisfied patients

- What type of equipment is used (archaic or state-of-the-art)

With the Internet and related technology, all of this can be done in the comfort of a patient's home. Dentistry does compete for discretionary income; however, an office does not want to compete on the basis of price. The real competitive advantage lies in creating value on the basis of convenience and service while minimizing costs. My caution to dental offices is to make sure you can deliver on the value you or your web site promises. Be responsive to your patients' needs, and they will sustain your referral base. Integrating the web with existing best-practice processes is not something that is set up once and forgotten; it is something that needs to be maintained and updated.

Computer-based oral health records are an electronic record and so can help to create a paperless office. Information can be transferred from general practitioner to specialist across the city or world for a second opinion. Documents can be electronically transferred to a medical office to ensure total health care and an interdisciplinary approach to treating the patient. Computers also offer decision support for treatment planning and patient assessment. A database that is easily accessible and regularly updated can provide an invaluable resource for care providers. The database is not the sole method of diagnosis, of course, but rather an aid in the decision-making process.

For example, technological advances in speech recognition will allow a practitioner to quickly produce a narrative to be shared with the patient or insurance company, based on his or her diagnosis. Speech recognition software can also be interfaced with practice management systems to allow importing of information from the patient's chart. This type of technology can be valuable in dictating letters, treatment planning, consultation, and/or diagnosis.

Computers used in education benefit both the patient and the professional. Increased use of interactive compact disc programs help reduce lag time between the introduction of new concepts and actual application. Databases containing dental literature can provide rapid access to current, specific information on dental treatments, products, and research. Patients can access information software in a dental office or via a modem, at home, in the areas of dentistry and dental hygiene that pertain to their needs or their families. In addition, an office can set up chat rooms or convenient ways for patients to ask questions and receive timely answers to enhance patient value.

Applications of structural capital to clinical and management data in dentistry and dental hygiene are increasing. As technology advances and computers become more recognized and accepted, dental practices will evolve into virtual health networks. Offices need to ensure that technology provides seamless pathways of information and integrated links for easy retrieval and input by professionals and patients.

Patient focus

Patient focus is the knowledge your practice has created through its relationships with its patients. This can be measured through patient referrals, patient-retention programs, or the percentage of patients who accept comprehensive care.

To build patient focus, a practice must share the office's knowledge with patients. Again, do not push this information on patients by stuffing their statement envelope with information about the newest whitening technique. Create knowledge links so that patients can browse for information on their own. Set up a database that patients can access, either at home or in your office, that outlines your policies, your suppliers, the specialists to whom you refer, the laboratories you use, and information about the staff, materials, standards, or whatever other knowledge your office has established.

Connect your patients to the experts—your knowledge teachers. Arrange informational nights in the office or chat sessions on the Internet to increase communication channels. Empower your patients with information about anything they want to discover—not what selected information you filter to them.

There are educational systems on the mass market that discuss procedures generally available in dentistry and dental hygiene. But your office controls the information flow. When a patient visits, the practitioner decides what procedures and what information is best for the patient to learn about. Why not allow the patient to access this information outside regular office hours? For example: On-line learning, where topics are categorized in lay terms, or 24-hour oral-health informational rooms.

As we establish ways for our patients to gain information from us, we also need to arrange a non-confrontational way to gain information from them. How are we serving their wants, what are their developing needs, what do they want us to provide for them? We need relationship feedback. We need to view our patients as a source of wealth for our practice—not only in the traditional sense of payment received for services rendered, but as information sources for future profitability. An office can gather these data, put them into a knowledge data bank, and allow its knowledge workers' creativity and innovation to build, mold, and provide the patient a solution-based service.

Professionalism: Definition and identification

So, how do *you* define professionalism in dentistry? Can you bridge the gaps between professionalism, profitability of the dental practice, and patient care? When professionalism is executed correctly and utilized efficiently, such initiatives ensure that all of a dental office's practices are best ones. Time isn't squandered on wheel reinvention, and valuable experience does not trail departing employees out the door—employees who were not versed in conflict resolution.

Of course, capturing *everything* a dental practice knows is probably impossible. So the first step in any "professionalism project" is to identify what knowledge pays the most to master.

- Do you want to improve your relationship with patients/ community?

- Build a more cohesive team?

- Make a transition to an aesthetic-enhancing restorative practice?

By identifying *what you have, what you use, what you need,* and *who should be responsible for it,* you will better understand and measure the professional process.

Identifying professional assets can also lead a practice to redefine its purpose, vision, and culture. These elements define why a practice is in business and ask what type of practice do we want to become? By analyzing a practice's unique assets of human capital, structural capital, and patient capital, we can determine its current and future capabilities. By examining its capabilities, after defining its values and purpose, an office can begin to develop short- and long-term knowledge strategies.

There are different types of professional knowledge. Building a knowledge-based organization may mean different things to different practices. For example, knowledge can be technical, behavioral, clinical, communicative, theory-based, and/or ethic-based. A practice that has determined that it has a strong core competency in periodontal treatments may also conclude that its interpersonal skills are less than ideal. It may decide that it needs to develop communication assets. Or a practice getting 15 new patients a month may determine that it has high behavioral knowledge; however, it needs to develop a computer-based intellectual asset in order to facilitate tracking and billing of patients.

Taking into account that the identification process within each office may take days, weeks, or hours, at some point in the future, all knowledge assets—if they truly have value—will convert into increased profitability. How can this be measured? Try assembling a "professional portfolio" or "professional report" (*i.e.,* Excel spreadsheet).

A professional report is a mechanism that allows an office to measure knowledge assets. A new technology for placing composite restorations or a new non-surgical management program, are examples of such assets. They may take months to develop and years to perfect, but at some point they must return revenues for the practice. An ancillary example may include development of indices and measurements for patient satisfaction, which in turn, may force the office to follow through for the sake of patient success measurements.

A written "scorecard" may raise the service bar that much higher and create effective intelligent practice-patient relations. It may identify a wrong technology or vendor, a lack of technological knowledge on the part of employees, or a service that is in conflict with the office philosophy. It may call for a reworking of office infrastructure or processes.

Measuring the human focus of a practice, though full of challenges, can help determine whether skills and expectations are aligned, where continuing development is desired, or if attributes exist in your office, untouched. These and other factors can systematically build a team member's development portfolio and professional program. As the professional assets are identified and developed, the measures change from investment and development to patient satisfaction, improved processes, increased referrals, and higher revenues and greater profits.

Building a professional base

Building an intellectual-based dental practice is not a one-time occurrence. The evolution starts and restarts with every reevaluation of the intellectual assets. This reevaluation may occur with a new employee, new service, a change in the competitive environment, or with new technologies. During the infancy stage, the knowledge manager/consultant needs to look for successes and publicize them, and work to make them become the best practices. As the knowledge process is continual, it does not always need to be a separate entity. To draw a parallel between knowledge practices and patient protection practices, when OSHA started to govern the dental profession and develop regulations, the new knowledge that accompanied the standards also brought a growth of new infection control consultants and experts. These experts educated your human capital, told you what structural capital you needed, and how to integrate it. However, as time and comfort increased, the OSHA standards of care become incorporated into every employee's workday. Practitioners now routinely perform the best practices of patient protection. Just as these infection-control principles have became second nature for practitioners, so will the aspects of intellectual capital.

Another predictive potential in building a professional report involves performing an audit of current structural capital, to determine index and prioritize target areas. General areas where practices can evaluate structural capital include cleaning up old paper and computer files and producing action lists, guidelines, or processes that can be duplicated and shared. Perhaps starting a customer database with value-added knowledge, codified. Posting and publicizing breakthrough ideas, blueprints on how-to procedures, lessons learned, or recent articles published in professional journals. Connect people to the data, and connect people to other individuals' tacit knowledge and expertise. Record team learning sessions so they may be retrieved when needed.

I caution that this does *not* mean pushing paper on people and making them sign off on them after a certain amount of time to make sure they have read them (whether or not it was retained or applied). This is about building and maintaining directories or storage bases where people can access the information when it is relevant to their current work situation.

Procedure manuals are a type of structural capital; but why not index them on computers and, instead of mandating that everyone read them and sign off that they did so during their first week of employment, allow employees to access them when they need certain policies, procedure updates, or restorative material information? Create a central database that houses the knowledge for the knowledge workers and the patient capital.

Dentistry and dental hygiene are changing more quickly than ever in response to new technologies, a vast increase in the amount of information, the ability to access that information, increased competition for providing dental/dental hygiene services, and the shift to knowledge work cultures. Compared to the job responsibilities most oral-health workers have been used to in the past, today's and tomorrow's jobs require a higher level of clinical skills, behavioral skills, and technological skills as well as knowledge creation and management.

Professionalism is packaged in the services and procedures we provide. It is packaged in the technologies we employ. The professionals in our offices allow us to sell convenience, flexibility, and a (hopefully) pleasant experience. Knowledge sharing applied to dentistry and dental hygiene provides us with a means of identifying those intangible factors, measuring them, and finding a way to provide better oral-health care and improving our patients' quality of life. It can also allow our patients to participate actively in their own treatment, which enhances the practitioner/patient relationship.

"The Need to Know..."

Validates your ability to achieve your professional goals and the practices goals. A written tracking report can identify gaps that may cause a team member to fall short of their goals and expectations.

Provides background information for re-evaluation for new services. When a new service is offered, racking will identify areas that must be met or developed.

Provides focus for education and training. Continuous education is the backbone of our professions, but few teams know what programs will actually enhance their productivity or value to the patient. An asset audit can help a professional team redesign its training decisions and attend programs that best meet these values.

Assess the value of the practice. Professional audits assess the intangible aspects of a person. Once identified and measured, they can be used in combination with the tangible assets to "grow" professionals and enhance their businesses.

Expands the practice's memory. The report can identify key assets and services so that the hygienist can properly use them. A team member can also recognize the professional "capital" he/she owns when preparing for a salary negotiation or a new dental "home".

Human Focus

- The average number of years of experience employees have in their professions
- Number of employee team members
- Team member turnover
- Leadership ability
- Motivation ability
- Empowerment ability
- Value added per employee

- Time in training (days/year)

- Are team members coachable?

- The percentage of patients who challenge the competencies of employees

- Among the many skills possessed by your team members, which do patients value most?

- Which skills and talents are most admired by your team members? What accounts for the difference between what patients value and what employees value?

- What percentage of team member time is spent in activity of low value to patients?

- What percent of producers' time is spent in activity of low value to patients?

- When competitors hire, do they hire from you?

- Why do people leave you to accept jobs elsewhere?

- What is your practice's reputation compared with other dental offices?

- Satisfied employee index

Structural Focus

- Administrative expense/total revenues

- Cost for administrative error processing time

- Administrative expense/employee

- IT capacity

- Change in IT inventory

- Structural capital development investment

- Suggestions made versus suggestions implemented. (If employees come up with 50 new ideas and the office only implements two of them, the structure may be hog-tying your people.)

- How long does it take to develop and educate staff in order to introduce new services?

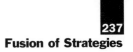

Client/Patient Focus

- Number of patients

- What is your patient retention (loyalty) rate?

- What is the increased (share of wallet) or work that is completed?

- Average duration of patient relationship

- Educational investment/patient

- Mechanism for patient feedback

- Patient rating/satisfied patient index

- Service of value to the patients.

Create Your Strategies

So much has been given me, I have no time to ponder that which had been denied • **Helen Keller**

This exercise, provided at the end of each chapter, is to assist you in designing a game plan to develop the skills, knowledge, and expertise necessary to propel you to your next level of personal and professional growth. Ask, answer, and record:

My distinctive team strategies for the future are:

_____

_____

_____

The areas for which I would like assistance and support to achieve my goals are:

_____

_____

_____

My action steps to get in the game and achieve those goals are:

_____

_____

_____

My list of specific goals and dates I wish to accomplish them includes:

_____

_____

_____

Possible obstacles to watch out for (i.e., fear of rejection, fear of change, and lack of accountability, denial, lack of focus, lack of self-evaluation, lack of mentoring relationships):

_____

_____

_____

APPENDIX I
Author and Contributors

Kristine A. Hodsdon, RDH, BS (Author)

Since 1989, Ms. Hodsdon has been changing the landscape of dentistry. She is editor with *Hygiene Mastery* news magazine, a hygiene coach, and international speaker. Kristine is a pioneer in the notion of connecting restorative dentistry with hygiene—and developed Pre-D Systems, a pre-diagnostic, computerized team checklist for comprehensive restorative and esthetic care. Her international seminars push, prod, and provoke participations to reinvent team roles and professionalism.

She is a regular columnist in *RDH* magazine and the *Journal of Cosmetic Dentistry*, and is a frequent contributor to dental industry publications, including *Dental Economics, Contemporary Oral Hygiene,* and *Dentistry Today*. She is a member of the ADHA and the AACD, served on the New Hampshire Board of Dental Examiners, and serves on several industry advisory councils and panels.

To reach Kristine about Pre-D Systems or her energetic programs, visit www.pre-dsystems.com or e-mail kahodsdon@pre-d.com

Bobbi Anthony, RDH

Ms. Anthony provides in-office consulting throughout the U.S. and Canada and has worked with more than 200 dental practices, offering a complete range of practice management and hygiene strategies to help them reach the next level of success. She also has been a part-time team instructor at LVI and the University of Southern California Periodontal Department. She can be contacted at bobbi@bobbianthony.com

Kristy Menage Bernie, RDH, BS

Ms. Menage Bernie was graduated with a BS degree and honors from the University of Maryland in 1984. In addition to clinical practice in pediatric, periodontic, and general practice settings, Kristy represented a major dental pharmaceutical company. Kristy owns a national meeting planning and consulting company, Educational Designs, which aids dental hygiene groups in formatting and managing continuing education courses, annual sessions, and securing corporate funding. Kristy serves as a featured columnist for *Contemporary Oral Hygiene* and has been a featured author on the topic of OSHA/CDC regulations, product innovations, full-mouth disinfection, and aesthetic/social enhancements. Kristy also lectures nationally on innovations in periodontal therapy, infection control and aesthetic dental hygiene. As an active member of the ADHA since graduation, Kristy has held numerous offices and volunteer positions over the years. She is the current President of the California Dental Hygienists' Association and is a Delegate to ADHA. Kristy may be contacted via e-mail at kmenageb@aol.com

Ann-Marie C. DePalma, RDH, BS

Ms. DePalma is a graduate of the Forsyth School for Dental Hygienists. She possesses a Bachelor of Health Science Degree from Northeastern University. Ann-Marie is active in the Massachusetts Dental Hygienists Association, having served in various positions, and is also a past president of the Forsyth Alumni Association. In 2000, she was awarded the Massachusetts Dental Society's Hygienist of the Year Award. Ann-Marie has been employed as a dental hygienist/surgical assistant in a periodontal office, and is employed as a clinical dental hygienist in a periodontal/implant practice. She is a certified instructor in the Dental Hygiene Implant Certification Program of the Association of Dental Implant Auxiliaries and Practice Management (a component of the International Congress of Oral Implantologists), a Fellow and Education and Membership Advisor of the ADIA &PM. Ann-Marie is also an educational consultant for Sulzer Dental,

Nobel Biocare, and 3i-Implant Innovations, leading implant manufacturers, with programs geared toward team members. She has written several articles for dental hygiene publications on dental implants. Ann-Marie has also lectured and written articles on TMD, with one article included in the NIH's National Oral Health Clearinghouses information packet on TMD. She is the founder of the TMJ Network, an educational resource for patients, as well as being involved in the TMJ Association, a national patient advocacy group. Ann-Marie has also developed a program for the dental team on recognizing childhood developmental delays. She is a Massachusetts Department of Public Health, Early Intervention Recertification Program parent member. She can be contacted at AMRDH@aol.com.

Deborah Dopson-Hartley, RDH

As a full-time practicing aesthetic hygienist of 25 years, Deborah Hartley, RDH lives and works her seminars everyday. She created and works a successful business, which not only increases her hygiene net profitability to over $100,00 per year, but also is instrumental in her ability to help influence and promote ideal comprehensive restorative and aesthetic dentistry. For more info, go to www.deborahhartley.com or call 813-985-5516

Jeffery Dornbush, DDS

Dr. Dornbush is known as the "best dentist on the North Shore" (Marblehead, Massachusetts), and his community regards him as an authority in all that dentistry has to offer.

Graduated from New York University College of Dentistry in 1975, Dr. Dornbush has developed many advances in dentistry in his interdisciplinary practice throughout his career. In 1976, he completed the Montefiore Hospital Internship Program under the directorship of Dr. Norman Treiger and Dr. Jack Kabcenell, who established the concepts of periodontal prosthesis. In 1978, Dr. Dornbush completed the two-year advanced graduate study in prosthodontics program at the Boston University School of Graduate Dentistry.

Dr. Dornbush has also become familiar with the protocols of restorative implant dentistry. He served as dental consultant and lecturer for Implant Innovations during its formative years in the early 1990s (the company was founded in 1987 by Dr. Richard

Lazzara and Dr. Keith D. Beaty in Palm Beach Gardens, Florida). Dr. Dornbush conducted a comprehensive hands-on course featuring the clinical application of dental implants in restorative dentistry both domestically and in Europe, and co-authored scholarly publications on the subject of interdisciplinary implant treatment in the *International Journal of Periodontics and Restorative Dentistry.*

Dr. Dornbush's affiliations include the Greater New York Academy of Prosthodontics; the Institute for Advanced Dental Studies (Swampscott); Aesthetic Advantage, Inc.; the Advanced Aesthetic Program at New York University, and the International College of Prosthodontists, The Northeastern Gnathological Society, the American Academy of Periodontics, the Academy of Osseointegration, Alpha Omega International Dental Fraternity, and the American Dental Association.

Most recently, Dr. Dornbush has dedicated himself to improving his patients' smiles through conservative, non-invasive cosmetic dental procedures, which have a positive impact on their overall appearance and self-confidence. His "smile makeovers" provide the patient a more youthful appearance through the implementation of procedures such as porcelain veneers, cosmetic bonding, and bleaching. In 1997, he became acquainted with the art of cosmetic dentistry at the Las Vegas Institute for Advanced Dental Studies. Beginning in September of that year, Dr. Dornbush became affiliated with Dr. Rosenthal's Aesthetic Advantage, Inc. a unique company dedicated to educating, motivating, and stimulating dental professionals.

Dr. Dornbush has immersed himself in understanding philosophies of occlusion—the Gnathological Approach; the Pankey-Mann Philosophy, and Neuromuscular Occlusion. Dr. Dornbush innovated "The Gold Occlusal Provisional Restoration" which provides a most stable occlusal position during the course of treatment. He gratefully acknowledges his working relationship with the technological talents of Advanced Dental Technologies and Jurium Dental Studio. He can be contacted via e-mail at dornbushj@attbi.com

Carol Jahn, R.D.H., MBA

Ms. Jahn has a BS in dental hygiene from the University of Iowa and an MS in continuing education and training management from the University of St. Francis, Joliet Il. She is employed as an Educational Representative by Waterpik Technologies, Inc, where she develops, promotes, and implements programs designed for the dental professional. Ms. Jahn is also a member of many editorial review boards. She may be contacted via e-mail at cjahn@waterpik.com

Carol Jent, RDH, MBA

Some people think that Carol Jent is trying to fit two lifetimes into one. When she wasn't running marathons, hunting big game, or crashing small planes in Alaska, she managed to obtain a degree in Dental Hygiene from the University of Alaska and later a degree in Communications and Marketing from the University of Utah. The two blend well in her position as Clinical Relations Manager for Ultradent where she works as a liaison between Ultradent and prominent clinician and organizations. She can be reached at dcarol@ultradent.com, www.ultradent.com

Kathleen Johnson

Founder and president of Kathleen Johnson and Associates (1993) and Aeropointe Management, Inc. (1988-1993), Kathleen has also worked as dental office assistant to administrators in private and multi-specialty practices.

She is the founder and lecturer for the Dental Management Study Club of Los Angeles/Orange County. As a certified instructor of private post-secondary education under California Education Code #94311, she has lectured at the U.C.L.A., School of Dentistry, Loma Linda University School of Dentistry, and has been an approved CE Provider for the California State Board of Dental Examiners since 1989, as well as an approved instructor for the state's Employment Training Program. Kathleen is also a member of the Dental Advisory Board of North-West College of Medical and Dental Assistants. She is a founding member of the board of the Academy of Dental Management Consultants, founded in 1989, and has been a member of the Protocol Foundation of Orange County since 1993

She has been published in the *Farran Report/DentalTown*, *Dental Business Today*, and the *ASDC Newsletter*. Her seminars include "Build the Practice You've Always Dreamed Of," "Reinventing Your Dental Practice Without Managed Care," "M & M's, Marketing and Management," "Maximizing Patient Flow, Retention, and Referral," "The Patient Visit Choreographed," "Creating a Patient Centered Practice," "Engineering the Ideal

Day," "Empowering the Dental Insurance Coordinator," and "Converting the Insurance Dependent Patient." She may be reached at kajohnson@sbcglobal.net

Trish Jones, RDH, BS

Ms. Jones is a technical advisor for Aurum Ceramic Dental Laboratories at the Las Vegas Institute for Advanced Dental Studies (LVI) in Las Vegas, Nevada. She assists dentists, hygienists, and team members in advanced laboratory communication in aesthetic dentistry. She also lectures to team members on behalf of JP Consultants Institute about aesthetic shade consulting, smile design, and post-care of the aesthetically restored smile.

Since earning her degrees (with honors) in dental hygiene and health care management from Southern Illinois University in Carbondale, Trish has been actively involved in the American Dental Hygienists Association. As a state delegate for Nevada and as a past president of Southern Nevada Dental Hygienists' Association, she participates in several community service projects. In 1999, she was presented the Outstanding Dental Hygienist Award from her local component.

She has maintained clinical practice for many years, as well as being adjunct clinical faculty at the Community College of Southern Nevada. She may be reached at trishj@aurumgroup.com or at 1-800-661-1169, Aurum Ceramic Dental Laboratories.

Jonathan B. Levine, DMD

A prosthodontist in private practice in New York City, Dr. Levine is clinical professor at NYU's Esthetics Department and Continuing Education Department. He is chairman and founder of DDS Partners, and may be reached at jlevine@ddspartners.com

Michael Maroon, DDS, FAGD

Dr. Maroon is editor and publisher of *The Dental Leader* newsletter (www.TheDentalLeader.com) and provides educational seminars through his Dental Dynamite! seminar series. He also is a co-founder of genR8TNext (Generation Next) seminars (www.genR8TNext.com) and moderates the genR8TNext dental e-mail network.

Dr. Maroon maintains an insurance–independent, aesthetic practice in Berlin, Conn. He is a member of the American Academy of Cosmetic Dentistry and the Crown Council.

For information, reach Dr. Maroon by phone at (860) 828-3933, by fax at (860) 828-1610, or by e-mail at drmikemaroon@aol.com.

Mary Martineau, RDH

Ms. Martineau, RDH, is a graduate of the dental hygiene program at Sacramento City College. She is a practicing dental hygienist and worked as a registered dental assistant for 14 years. She received her standard proficiency certificate for the diode laser in 1998 and currently teaches laser soft tissue curettage at the Center for Advanced Dentistry in Los Angeles.

Ms. Martineau lectures regularly and has published articles on the use of lasers in dental hygiene. She owns and operates High-Tech Hygiene, a coaching program for hygienists. She can be contacted at maryanrdh@aol.com or via www.laserhygieneconsulting.com.

Vicki McManus, RDH

Ms. McManus, RDH, is director of Hygiene Mastery, an in-office coaching program developed to address the unique clinical and business challenges within the hygiene department. She is also a business coach with Fortune Management, a faculty member of the prestigious Pacific Aesthetic Continuum (PAC~Live) in San Francisco, and is the collaborative author of *FUNdamentals of Outstanding Dental Teams*.

She has been published in *Dentistry Today, Dental Economics, The Profitable Dentist, and Contemporary Oral Hygiene* and is editor of a new publication the *Hygiene Mastery Newsmagazine*. This innovative magazine's main goal is to offer a median connecting the doctor and hygienists and assistants. She is a featured speaker at PAC-Live, Yankee Dental Congress, The Profitable Dentist Spring Break in Destin, and Tony Robbins' Personal Power Seminars for Dentistry.

To reach Vicki and receive a complimentary analysis of your hygiene department's potential, call (888) 347-4785, email vicki@hygienemastery.com, or write:

Hygiene Mastery, Fortune Management

5579-B Chamblee Dunwoody Road, Suite 207

888.347.4785/ f. 770.512.0892

Lynn D. Terracciano-Mortilla, RDH

Ms. Terracciano-Mortilla is a practicing clinical dental hygien-ist in Tarpon Springs, Florida. Her studies and work with implants began shortly after her licensure from the dental hygiene pro-gram at the State University of New York at Farmingdale. She became involved with the International Congress of Oral Implantologists in 1995 and is the executive director of their aux-iliary section, the Association of Dental Implant Auxiliaries & Practice Management (ADIA & PM). She has been involved with the dental hygiene implant certification program since its cre-ation in 1995.

She is a fellow of the ADIA & PM/ICOI and a member of the continuing education faculty at the University of Texas Health Science Center in San Antonio. Lynn lectures internationally and publishes on dental implants, maintenance concerns, and proce-dures involving dental implants. Her goal is to educate and involve all members of the implant team on the verbal and inter-disciplinary skills needed to have a successful and profitable implant practice. She can be reached at (813) 304-2637 or email: LDTRDH@aol.com.

Trisha E. O'Hehir, RDH, BS

Ms. O'Hehir received degrees in dental hygiene and higher education at the University of Minnesota. More than 30 years as a dental hygienist have included private practice in the United States and Zurich, Switzerland, and faculty positions at the uni-versities of Minnesota, Washington, and Arizona. She pioneered the position of periodontal therapist in Arizona and worked for several years teaching local anesthesia and providing local anes-thesia in an oral surgery practice.

In addition to extensive clinical practice experience, she is an international lecturer, consulting editor for *RDH Magazine*, editor of *Perio Reports Newsletter*, and co-founder of the Perio-Data Company. She has authored the textbook, *Compendium of Current Research*, contributed to the texts *Comprehensive Dental*

Hygiene Care by Irene Woodall, and *Comprehensive Periodontics for the Dental Hygienist* by Dr. Mea Weinberg. Her articles have appeared in *RDH, JDH, JPH, Access,* and *JADA.* She is a member of many North American professional organizations, such as the International Academy of Periodontology, International Federation of Dental Hygienists, and the International Association for Dental Research.

Her awards include the 1991 Distinguished Alumni Award from the University of Minnesota School of Dental Hygiene and the Warner-Lambert/ADHA Excellence in Dental Hygiene Award. Trisha currently lives and works in Arizona, where she is a past president of the Arizona State Dental Hygienists' Association. She is considered a future-focused thinker who presents thought-provoking programs combining current research, practical applications, and alternatives for the future. Contact her at (520) 374-4290 or (800)-374-4290 or at

www.PerioReports.com or trisha@PerioReports.com

Tricia Osuna, RDH, BS

Ms. Osuna received a Bachelor of Science degree in dental hygiene from the School of Dentistry, University of Southern California in 1978. She was in clinical practice in the Los Angeles area until July 2001. She has recently completed her fourth year as the dental hygienist representative on the USC Dental Alumni Association board of directors. In addition to private practice, Tricia was a clinical instructor at the UCLA School of Dentistry in the department of advanced general dentistry.

Professionally, Tricia has been quite active in her association since graduation, serving as an elected delegate to the annual sessions of the Southern California Dental Hygienists Association, the California Dental Hygienists' Association, and the American Dental Hygienists Association. Tricia has also served as president of the South Bay Dental Hygienists Society and in numerous positions in both the Los Angeles and South Bay Dental Hygienists Societies. In 1992, she was elected to a term as President of the California Dental Hygienists Association.

Recognized for her many efforts and contributions to the dental hygiene profession, Tricia has received several awards, including the CDHA's President's Recognition Award and the ADHA Bausch and Lomb "Distinctions in Dental Hygiene" Award.

Tricia's company, Professional Insights, provides consulting services and market research evaluations on dental and dental hygiene products to companies worldwide. She is currently providing consulting services in the position of Corporate Relations Consultant for the California Dental Hygienists Association and is a newly appointed member of the California Board of Dental Examiners. She can be reached at osunardh@aol.com

Maria Perno Goldie, RDH, MS

A professional member of the National Speakers Association, Maria was graduated from the University of Pennsylvania, School of Dental Hygiene in 1971 and is the recipient of the 1999 University of Pennsylvania Dental Hygiene Alumni Achievement Award. She earned her BA in health services administration from Saint Mary's College in Moraga, CA, and an MS in Health Science from San Francisco State University.

As a noted researcher, author, and speaker, Maria has presented seminars nationally and internationally on topics such as Women's Health and Wellness, Oral Care for the Cancer Patient, Oral Cancer, and Immunology and Periodontal Disease. She has appeared in several network television interviews regarding the link between periodontal disease and systemic disease.

Maria served as the 1997-98 President of the American Dental Hygienists' Association (ADHA). She is a member of the International Association for Dental Research (IADR), Oral Health Research Group, the American Dental Education Association (ADEA), and is an American Dental Hygienists Association (ADHA) delegate to the International Federation of Dental Hygienists (IFDH). Maria is a life member of the ADHA and the California Dental Hygienists' Association (CDHA).

Maria was appointed to the National Women's Health Resource Center (NWHRC) Women's Health Advisory Council, and reviews content for their website. She is on the advisory board of Dental X-Change, the largest commercial dental Internet Web site. As an active board member of the Dental Health Foundation, the dental public health organization in California, she helps underserved communities and contributes to the education and policy-making of a number of organizations.

Reach her at http://www.seminarsforwomenshealth.com or mariaperno1@attbi.com

Jill Rethman, RDH, BA

Ms. Rethman has more than 20 years of experience in dental hygiene. A graduate of Ohio State University, she has practiced in both general and periodontal settings. Currently, she works as a consultant to the dental industry, designing educational programs.

Jill has presented programs to dental and dental hygiene societies, dental schools, and study clubs and associations throughout the United States, Canada, Europe, and Japan. Topics include periodontal updates, ultrasonic instrumentation, geriatric patient considerations, patient compliance and communication, and new product reviews.

Her articles have been featured in the *Journal of the American Dental Association, Journal of Practical Periodontics and Aesthetic Dentistry,* and *Dentistry Today.* Jill is the editor-in-chief of the *Journal of Practical Hygiene.* She was recently appointed to the American Academy of Periodontology's Task Force on Dental Hygiene Education, and has co-authored a chapter for the textbook *Comprehensive Periodontics for the Dental Hygienist.*

A consultant to the ADA's Future of Dentistry Project, Jill is a visiting clinical instructor at the University of Pittsburgh, School of Dental Medicine, Department of Dental Hygiene, and is a featured speaker for the American Dental Association's Seminar Series.

She can be reached at grethman@hotmail.com or www.JillRethman.com.

Allison Roberts, EFDA

Ms. Roberts, an expanded-function dental assistant (EFDA), is Deborah Hartley's aesthetic hygiene assistant. She can be reached at www.deborahartley.com

Donna M. Sirvydas, RDH, M.Ed.

Ms. Sirvydas was a full-time clinical hygienist for 12 years before returning to school to pursue undergraduate work in psychology and her graduate degree in school counseling. She currently works as the guidance director at Presentation of Mary Academy (PMA), a private Catholic school for grades K-8, while still holding her active hygiene license in two states. She can be reached at sirvydas@mymailstation.com

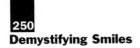

Karen Stueve, RDH

Ms. Stueve grew up in Ottawa, Ohio, and was graduated from Lima (OH) Technical College with a degree in dental hygiene. She currently practices dental hygiene in Minster, in west central Ohio.

She has been a member of ADHA since 1996, and works "in a wonderful, high quality, preventive-oriented practice." She can be reached at jkstueve@nktelco.net

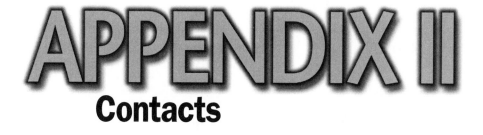
APPENDIX II
Contacts

3M ESPE Dental Products
3M Center, Building 275-2SE-03
St. Paul, MN 55144-1000
1-800-634-2249
www.3MESPE.com

American Academy of Cosmetic Dentistry
2810 Walton Commons West, Suite 200
Madison, WI 53718
800-543-9220
fax: 608-222.9540
www.aacd.com
info@aacd.com

American Academy of Esthetic Dentistry
401 N. Michigan Ave.
Chicago, IL 60611
312-321-5121
Fax: 312-673-6953
aaed@sba.com
www.estheticacademy.org

American Dental Assistant's Association

203 North LaSalle Street. Suite 1320

Chicago, IL 60601

312-541-1550

Fax: 312-541-1496

American Dental Hygienists' Association

444 N. Michigan Ave., Suite 3400

Chicago, IL 60611

800-243-2342

Fax: 312-467-1806

www.adha.org

Association of Dental Implant Auxiliaries and Practice Management

248 Lorraine Avenue, Third Floor

Upper Montclair, NJ 07043-1454

973.783.6300

Fax: 973.783.1175

www.dentalimplants.com/ icoi@dentalimplants.com

For more information about ADIA & PM:

Ann-Marie C. DePalma, RDH, BS, AMRDH@aol.com

Lynn D. Terracciano- Mortilla, RDH, ADIA & PM executive director, LDTRDH@aol.com

Aurum Ceramic Dental Laboratories

1320 N. Howard

Spokane, WA 99201-2412

1-800-661-1169

www.aurumgroup.com/ -E-MAIL: cerum@aurumgroup.com

Biolase Technology, Inc.

981 Calle Amanecer

San Clemente, CA 92673

888.4.BIOLASE

www.biolase.com

Butler

John O. Butler Company

4635 W. Foster Avenue

Chicago, IL 60630

www.jbutler.com

CAESY Education System

1201 SE Tech Center Drive, Suite 110

Vancouver, WA 98683

800-691-1980

www.caesy.com

CollaGenex Pharmaceuticals Inc.

21031 Monisha

Lake Forest, CA 92630-6425

www.collagenex.com

Dawson Center for Advanced Dental Study

Masters Library Series

111 Second Avenue, NE, Suite 1109

St. Petersburg, FL 33701

Fax: (843) 406.7617

www.dawsncenter.com

Dental Economics Magazine

Box 3408

Tulsa, OK 74101

(800) 633-1681

Editor: Joseph A. Blaes, DDS

joeb@pennwell.com

DentalView

34-B Mauchly Street

Irvine, CA 92618-2357

www.dentalview.com

DENTSPLY Professional Division

1301 Smile Way, P O Box 7807

York, PA 17404-0807

(800) 989-8826 Customer Service

www:dentsply.com

Discus Dental

8550 Higuera St.

Culver City, CA 90232

800-422-9448

Fax: 310-845-1500

www.discussdental.com

Hu-Friedy

3232 North Rockwell Street

Chicago, IL 60618-5935

800.HU.FRIEDY

www.hu-friedy.com

Hygiene Mastery

5579-B Chamblee Dunwoody Road

Suite #207

Atlanta, GA 30338

888.347.4785

www.hygienemastery.com

Ivoclar Vivadent

175 Pineview Drive

Amherst, NY 14228

800.553.6825

www.ivoclarvivadent.us.com

Paul Homoly, DDS & Associates

127 West Worthington Avenue Suite 200

Charlotte, NC 28203

704.342.4900.9370

704.342.4995-fax

www.paulhomoly.com/ paul@paulhomoly.com

Philips Oral Healthcare, Inc.

35301 SE Center Street

Snoqualmie, WA 98065

425-396-2000/ 800-676-Sonic

www.sonicare.com

Premier Dental

3600 Horizon Drive

Box 61574

King of Prussia, PA 19406-0974

888.773.6872

www.premusa.com

International Federation of Dental Hygienists

55 Kemble Road, Forest Hill

London SE 23 2DH. UK

+44-208-699-3531

f: +44 208-488-1067

Laclede, Inc., Healthcare Products Division

2030 East University Drive

Rancho Dominguez, CA 90220

(310) 605-4280

Fax: (310) 605-4288

www.laclede.com

Las Vegas Institute For Advanced Dental Studies

9501 Hillwood

Las Vegas, NV 89134

(702) 341-7978

(702) 341-8510 fax

www.lvilive.com

MicroDental Laboratories

5601 Arnold Road

Dublin, CA 94568

800.229.0936

www.microdental.com

Omnii Oral Pharmaceuticals

1500 North Florida Mango Road, Suite 1

West Palm Beach, FL 33409-5208

800.445.3386

www.omniipharma.com

Oral B Laboratories

600 Clipper Dr.

Belmont, CA 94002-4119

800.446.7252.

Fax: 650.591.3396

www.oralb.com

OraPharma, Inc.

732 Louis Drive

Warminster, PA 18974

p. 215.956.2235

f. 215.443.9531

www.orapharma.com

Oxyfresh

Anthony Stefanou, DMD

Divisional Leader, Dental Care

Corporate Offices

12928 East Indiana Avenue

Spokane, WA 99216

Voicemail: 800.999.9551 ext. 352

oxytony@aol.com

Pacific Aesthetic Continuum

Pac~Live

San Francisco, CA

(310) 845-8340

PracticeWorks/Dicom

1765 The Exchange

Atlanta, GA 303339

770-850-5006

www.practiceworks.com

RDH Magazine

Box 3408

Tulsa, OK 74101

(800) 633-1681

Editor: Mark Hartley

MarkH@Pennwell.com

Reality Publishing Co.

11757 Katy Freeway, Suite 210

Houston, TX 77079-1717

800.544.4999

Fax: 281.493.1558

www.realityesthetics.com

SDS/Kerr

1717 W. Collins Ave.

Orange, CA 92867

800.537.7123

www.kerrdental.com

Shofu Dental Corporation

1225 Stone Drive

San Marcos, CA 92069-4059

1-800-82-SHOFU

www.shofu.com

Sultan Chemist

85 W. Forest Ave.

Englewood, NJ 07631

800-637-8582/ 201-871-1232

Fax: 201.871.0321

www.sultanintl.com

Tekscan, Inc.

307 West First Street

South Boston, MA 02127-1309

800.248.3669

www.tekscan.com

Water Pik Technologies

Personal Healthcare Products

1730 E. Prospect Rd.

Fort Collins, CO 80553

www.waterpik.com

Ultradent

505 W. 10200 S.

South Jordan, UT 84095

800.552.5512/ 801.572-4200

Fax; 801.572.0600

www.ultradent.com

Young Dental

13705 Shoreline Court East

Earth City, MO 63045

800-325-1881

Fax: 866-GO-YOUNG

www.youngdental.com

REFERENCES

Understanding The Bigger Picture

Chapter 1

Condon, J.R., Francine K.L., "Assessing the effect of composite formulation on polymerization stress," *Journal of the American Dental Association*, 131 April 497-503, 2000.

Dawson P.E., *Diagnosis, management, and treatment of temporomandibular disorders.* (position paper) American Equilibration Society to NIDR, NIH 1996:1-4.

Esquivel-Upshaw, Josephine F., Anusavice, Kenneth J., Reid, Megan, Yang, Mark C.K., Lee, Robert B., "Fracture resistance of all-ceramic and metal ceramic inlays," *International Journal of Prosthodontics*, 2001:14(2):109-114.

Fortin, D, Vargas, M.A., "The spectrum of computers: new technologies and materials," *Journal of the American Dental Association*, June 26s-30s, 2000.

Fradeani, M., Aquilano, A., "Clinical experience with Empress crowns," *International Journal of Prosthodontics*, 1997:10(3): 241-247.

Frankenberger, R., Petschelt, A., Kramer, N., "Leucite-reinforced glass ceramic inlays and onlays after six years: Clinical behavior," *Operative Dentistry 2000.* 25:459-465.

Klaff, David, BDS, blending incremental and stratified layering techniques to produce an esthetic posterior composite resin restoration with a predictable prognosis," *Journal of Esthetic Restorative Dentistry* 13: 101-113, 2001.

Ludwig, K., Dr., "Studies on the ultimate strength of all ceramic crowns," *Dental Labor* No.5:647-651, 1991.

Mange, P., "Conservative restoration of compromised posterior teeth with direct composites: A seven-year report." *Practical Periodontal Aesthetic Dentistry* 12, (8)2000,p. 747-749.

O'Brien, W.J., "Strengthening mechanisms of current dental porcelains," *Compendium of Continuing Education in Dentistry* 21 625-630, 2000.

Ritter, Andre V., "Posterior resin-based composite restorations: clinical recommendations for optimal success," *Journal of Esthetic Restorative Dentistry*, 13 2001, p. 88-99.

Telles D, Pegoraro, L.F., Pereira, J.C., "Prevalence of noncarious cervical lesions and their relation to occlusal aspects: A clinical study," *Journal of Esthetic Dentistry 2000* 12 (1): 10-15, 2000.

Chapter 2

Cehreli, Z.C., Altay, N., "Three-year clinical evaluation of a polyacid-modified resin composite in minimally-invasive occulsal cavities," *Journal of the American Dental Association,* February 2000: 117-122.

Croll, T.P., "Enamel microabrasion: observations after 10 years," *Journal of the American Dental Association* 1997 Apr; 128 Suppl: 45S-50S

Croll, T.P., "Tooth bleaching for children and teens: a protocol and examples." *Quintessence International* 1994 Dec; 25(12): 811-7.

Darby, Michele, Walsh, Margaret M., *Dental Hygiene Theory and Practice,* W.B. Saunders Company, Philadelphia, 1995: 15-45

Ibid, pps. 47-55, 327-359.

Dawson Center for Advanced Dental Study, *Master Library Series,* St Petersburg, FL 1998.

de Araujo, F.B., Zis, V, Dutra, C.A.V., "Enamel color change by microabrasion and resin-based composite." *Journal of the American Dental Association.* 1999; 13 (1): 6-7.

Erdogan, G, "The effectiveness of a modified hydrochloric acid-quartz-pumice abrasion technique on fluorosis stains: a case report," *Quintessence International* 1998 Feb; 29(2): 119-22.

Garber, David A., "Increased application of digital radiography for implant therapy." *Practical Periodontics & Aesthetic Dentistry;* January/February 2000, Volume 12 No.1: 73-74.

Golub-Evans, Jeffery, "A short history of smile design," *Contemporary Esthetics and Restorative Practice,* February 1999; 70-73.

Hodsdon, Kristine, "Postoperative care for aesthetic restorations: A challenge to dental hygienists," *Journal of Practical Hygiene* March/April 1998; 19-24.

Isler, S., "Esthetic principles; concepts, and practices in pediatric and adolescent dentistry," *Dental Clinicians of North America,* 1989 Apr; 33(2): 171-81

Kehoe, Bob, "Working amalgam-free: The moment of truth," *Dental Practice & Finance,* September/October 1998: 25-34.

Levin, Roger P., "Increasing cosmetic patient motivation," *The Journal of Cosmetic Dentistry,* Volume 13, (3) Fall 2000: 45-47

Linder, Annette Ashley, RDH, "Hygiene check will build your practice," *Dental Practice & Finance,* September/October 1998: 57-60.

Okeson, Jeffrey P., *Management of Temporomandibular Disorders and Occlusion, 4th edition.,* St. Louis, Mosby 1998.

McGuire, Michael K., Miller, Lynn,. "Maintaining esthetic restorations in the periodontal practice," *International Journal of Periodontal & Restorative Dentistry* 1996; Vol. 16, No. 3: 231-239.

Miller, M.B., *Reality Publishing Co.,* Houston: January 2000; Volume 4.

Mohl/Zarb/Carlsson/Rugh, *A Textbook of Occlusion,* Chicago, Quintessence Publishing Co., Inc., 1991.

Narcisi, Edward M., DMD, DiPerna, James A., DMD, "Multidisciplinary full-mouth restoration with porcelain veneers and laboratory-fabricated resin inlays." *Practical Periodontal Aesthetic Dentistry* 1999; 11 (6): 721-728.

Nash, Linda, "Improving aesthetics with porcelain laminate veneers." *Journal of Practical Hygiene,* May/June 1996; 21-25.

Nash, Linda, "The hygienist's role in aesthetic and cosmetic restorations," *Journal of Practical Hygiene* 1994; 3 (3); 9-12.

Roth, Sandra R., *ProSpective, Volume One: Reclaiming the Passion of Dentistry,* ProSynery Press, Seattle Washington, p. 1-20. 1993.

Roth, Sandra, R., *ProSpective, Volume Two: Defining the Mission of Dentistry,* ProSynery Press, Seattle Washington p. 73-92. 1995.

Wells, Dennis J, DDS, "The lateral incisor: The unsung hero in smile design," *AACD Journal,* Fall 1999:38-46.

Woodall, Irene, Ph.D., RDH, "Do not let the changes in dental hygiene pass you by," *RDH Magazine,* Febuary 1990: 6-7.

Chapter 3

Axellson, P., "An introduction to risk prediction and preventive dentistry," unpublished.

Dean, H.T., Arnold. F.A., Jr., Elove, E., *Domestic water and dental caries, V:* "Additional studies of the relation of fluoride domestic waters to dental caries experience in 4425 white children aged 12-14 years in 13 cities in four states," *Public Health Reports,* 57:1155-1179.

Garcia-Godoy, F., Hicks, M. J., Flaitz, C., Berg, J., "Acidulated phosphate fluoride treatment and formation of caries-like lesions in enamel: Effect of application time," *Journal of Clinical Pediatric Dentistry,* 19: 2 1995.

Hicks, M.J., Flaitz, C.M., "Epidemiology of dental caries in the pediatric and adolescent population: a review of past and current trends," *Journal of Clinical Pediatric Dentistry*, 18:43-50,1993.

Hodsdon, Kristine, "Postoperative care for aesthetic restorations: A challenge to dental hygienists," *Journal of Practical Hygiene,* March/April 1998; 19-24.

Ogaard, B., Rolla, G., Dijkman, T., Ruben, J., Arends, Jet, "Effect of fluoride mouthrinsing on caries lesions in development of shark enamel: An in situ model study," *Scandinavian Journal of Dental Restorations,* (1999) 99:372-377.

Ogaard, B., Seppa, L., Rolla, G., "Professional topical fluoride applications: clinical efficacy and mechanism of action," *Advance Dental Restorations,* 8(2):190-201, July 1994.

Soeno/Matsumura/Atsuta/Kawasaki, "Effect of acidulated phosphate flouride solution on veneering particulate filler composite," *The International Journal of Prosthodontics,* Volume 14, Number 2, p.127-132, 2001.

Soeno/Matsumura/Kawasaki/Atsuta, "Influence of acidulated phosphate fluoride agents on the surface characteristics of composite restorative materials," *American Journal of Dentistry*, Vol. 13, No.6 297-300, December 2000.

Soeno/Matsumura/Kawasaki/Atsuta, "Influence of acidulated phosphate fluoride agents and effectiveness of subsequent polishing on composite material surfaces," *Operative Dentistry*, 27, 305-310, 2002.

Wilkins, Esther M., *Clinical practice of the dental hygienist, 8th ed.,* 1999.

Chapter 4

American Academy of Periodontology Position Paper: Periodontal Disease as a Potential Risk Factor for Systemic Diseases. *Journal of Clinical Periodontology,* 1998; 841 – 849.

"American Dental Hygienists' Association policy definitions," *Optimal Oral Health · 1999*

Ahmad, Irfan, BDS, "Geometric consideration in anterior dental esthetics: restorative principles," *Practical Periodontal Aesthetic Dentistry_1998; 10 (7): 813-822.*

Armitage, G.C., "Development of a classification system for periodontal disease and conditions," *Ann Periodontal,* Vol. 4 · Number 1 · December, 1999.

Bader, H., "Floss or die: Implications for dental professionals," *Dentistry Today* 1998; July.

Bollen, C.M.L., Vandekerckhove, B.N.A., Papaioannou W., *et. al.:* "Full- versus partial-mouth disinfection in the treatment of periodontal infections: Long term microbiological observations," *Journal of Clinical Periodontology,* 1996; 23: 960 – 970.

Bollen, C.M.L., Vandekerckhove, B.N.A., Papaioannou W., *et. al.:* "The effect of a full-mouth disinfection on different intraoral niches: Clinical and microbiological observations," *Journal of Clinical Periodontology,* 1998; 25: 56 – 66.

Bosy, A., Kulkarni, G.V., Rosenberg, M., McCullough, C.A.G., "Relationship of oral malodor to periodontitis: Evidence of independence in discrete subpopulations, *Journal of Clinical Periodontology,* 1994; 65(1): 37 – 46.

Bray, K.K., Wilder, R.S., "Full-mouth disinfection: A new approach to non-surgical periodontal therapy," *Access* September – October 1999; 57 – 60.

Cancro, L.P. & Fishcman, S.L., "The expected effect on oral health of dental plaque control through mechanical removal," *Periodontology 2000* Vol. 8, 1995 : 60 – 74.

Caton, J., Ciancio, S., Crout, R., *et. al.:* "Treatment with subantimicrobial dose doxycycline improves the efficacy of scaling and root planing in patients with adult periodontitis," *Periodontology 2000* Vol. 71 (4): 521 – 532.

Center for Disease Control and Prevention: Recommendations for Using Fluoride to Prevent and Control Dental Caries in the United States, MMWR 2001, Vol. 50 (RR-14) – August 17, 2001.

Christensen G., "Why clean your tongue?" *Journal of the American Dental Association,* 1998; 129 (11): 1605 – 1607.

Clark, G., Nachnani, S., Messadi, D., "Detecting and treating oral and non-oral malodor," *Journal of the California Dental Association* 1997; 25(2): 133 – 143.

Dietschi, Diadier, DMD, "A century of operative dentistry," *Practical Periodontics & Aesthetic Dentistry,* January/February 2000, Volume 12 No.1: 92-93.

Ditolla, Michael C., DDS, "Practice builders: esthetic periodontics," *Contemporary Esthetics and Restorative Dentistry,* July/August 1999, 22.

Drisko, C., "Non-surgical periodontal therapy," *Periodontology 2000* 2001; 25: 77 – 88.

Eickholz, P., Kim, T.S., Burklin, T., *et. al.*: "Non-surgical periodontal therapy with adjunctive topical doxycycline: a double-blind randomized controlled multicenter study (I); Study design and clinical results." *Journal of Clinical Periodontology,* Vol. 29 (2): 108 – 117.

Garrett, S., Johnson, L., Drisko, C., *et. al.*: "Two multi-center studies evaluating locally delivery doxycycline hyclate, placebo control, oral hygiene and scaling and root planing in the treatment of periodontitis," *Journal of Periodontology* 1999; 70 (5): 490 – 503.

Lazarus, Jan, Sprague, Peggy, "Revolutionary adjunctive treatment modalities," *LVI- Dental Visions.* March/April Volume 9, Number 2,18-19.

Narcisi, Edward M., DMD, DiPerna, James A., DMD, "Multidisciplinary full-mouth restoration with porcelain veneers and laboratory-fabricated resin inlays," *Practical Periodontal Aesthetic Dentistry 1999*; 11 (6): 721-728.

Robbins, William J., DDS, MA, "Dental diagnosis and treatment of excessive gingival display," *Practical Periodontal Aesthetic Dentistry 1999*; 11 (2): 265-272.

Rosenthal, Larry, DDS, Jacobs, James E., DMD, "The periodontal-prosthetic-esthetic connection," *Contempory Esthetics and Restorative Practice,* July/August 1999: 12-16.

Takei, Henry H., DDS, MS, *et. al.*, "Surgical crown lengthening of the maxillary anterior dentition: aesthetic consideration," *Practical Periodontal Aesthetic Dentistry 1999*; 11 (5): 639-644.

Chapter 5

Cheek, Caroline, Heyman, Harold O., DDS, Med., "Dental and oral discoloration associated with minocycline and other tetracycline analogs," *The Journal of Esthetic Dentistry,* Volume 11, Number 1.p.43-48.

Chung, S.M., Kim, W.J., "Effect of tooth bleaching agents on color restorative materials" (abstract 1127) and Saito, Y., Toko, T., *et.al.:* "Effect of peroxide on color stability of newly fabricated or 1-year-old restorative materials" (abstract 1128), *Journal of Dental Restorations 2000*, 79 (special issue); 284.

Crispin, Bruce J., DDS., MS., "Literature review," *American Academy of Cosmetic Dentistry Journal,* Winter 1999; pp. 6-7.

Department of Diagnostic Science & General Dentistry, *CB #7450,* University of North Carolina, Chapel Hill, NC 27599-740; Carolyn_Bentley@dentistry.unc.edu.

Engelhardt, Debra, "Practice builders: Whiter smiles." *Contemporary Esthetics and Restorative Practice Vol. 3,* No 5, pp. 48; May 1999.

Gokay, Osman, DDS, *et. al.,* "Penetration of the pulp chamber by bleaching agents in teeth restored with various restorative materials," *Journal of Endodontics* Volume 26, Number 2 February 2000.

Goldstein, Ronald, DDS, "Tooth whitening in your practice: Treatment time and fee schedules," *Contemporary Esthetics and Restorative Practices,* November/December 2000. p. 12-15.

Hansen, P.A., Killoy, W., Masterson, K., "Effect of brushing with sonic and counter-rotational toothbrushes on the bond strength of orthodontic brackets," *American Journal of Orthodontics and Dentofacial Orthopedics,* Vol.115, No.1, Jan 1999, pp.55-60.

Haywood B., "Historical development of whiteners clinical safety and efficacy." *Oral Health,* pp. 27-37, April 1999.

Hodsdon, Kristine, "Post-operative care for aesthetic restorations: A challenge to dental hygienists," *Journal of Practical Hygiene* March/April 1998, 19-24.

Javaheri, D.S., Janis J.N., "The Efficacy of reservoirs in bleaching trays," *Operative Dentistry,* Volume 25, Number 3, May/June 2000.

Jones, Aaron H., Diaz-Arnold, M., Anna, "Colorimetric assessment of laser and home beaching techniques," *Journal of Esthetic Dentistry Volume 11, Number 2,* pp. 87-94,1999.

Kugel, G, Non-tray whitening, *Compendium of Continuing Education in Dentistry 2000,* 21 (6): 524-528.

Kula, K., McKinney, J., Kula, T., "Effects of daily topical fluoride gels on resin composite degradation and wear," *Dental Materials,* Vol. 13, No.5 Sept. 1997, pp.305-311.

Leonard, Ralph H., *et.al.,* "Nightguard vital bleaching of tetracycline-stained teeth: 54 months post treatment," *Journal of Esthetic Dentistry,* Volume 11, Number 5 p. 265-277.

Levine, A., and Robert and Richard Shanaman, "translating clinical outcomes to patient value: An evidence-based treatment approach," *The International Journal of Periodontics & Restorative Dentistry,* Volume 15, Number 2, pp. 187-200, April 1995.

Matis, Bruce, "In vivo degradation of bleaching gel used In whitening teeth," *Journal of the American Dental Association,* Vol. 130, pp. 227-235. February 1999.

McGuire, Michael K., Miller, Lynn, "Maintaining esthetic restorations in the periodontal practice," *International Periodontal Restorative Dentistry* 1996; 16:231-239.

Meltser, Lynn, "The dental hygienists' role in patient home-care motivation," *Access Special Supplemental Issue,* pp. 1-12, April 1999.

Miller, M.B., *Maintaining Esthetic Restorations,* Houston: Reality Publishing Co. Volume 14, Section 3; 237-248.

Nash Linda, "Improving aesthetics with porcelain laminate veneers," *Journal of Practical Hygiene* May/June 1996; 21-25.

Nash, Linda, "The hygienist's role in aesthetic and cosmetic restorations," *Journal of Practical Hygiene* 1994; 3 (3); 9-12.

Oliver, Trudy L., RDH, MS, Haywood, Van B. DMD, "Efficacy of nightguard vital bleaching technique beyond the borders of a shortened tray," *Journal Of Esthetic Dentistry,* Volume 11, Number 2, p. 95-102.

Rethman, Jill, "Tooth whitening: Stains and their origins," *The Journal of Practical Hygiene: Special Whitening Supplement,* Volume 7, Number 4, pp. 38-39, 1999.

Soeno/Matsumura/Atsuta/Kawasaki, "Effect of acidulated phosphate flouride solution on veneering particulate filler composite," *The International Journal of Prosthodontics*, Volume 14, Number 2, p.127-132, 2001.

Soeno/Matsumura/Kawasaki/Atsuta, "Influence of acidulated phosphate fluoride agents on the surface characteristics of composite restorative materials," *American Journal of Dentistry*, Volume 13, No.6 297-300, December 2000.

Soeno/Matsumura/Kawasaki/Atsuta, "Influence of acidulated phosphate fluoride agents and effectiveness of subsequent polishing on composite material surfaces," *Operative Dentistry*, 27, 305-310, 2002.

Swift, E.J., Predigao, J., "Effects on bleaching on teeth and restoration," Special Issue on Nightguard Bleaching, Paper d, 815-820.

Swift J., Edward, Kenneth, N. May, "Two-year clinical evaluation of tooth whitening using an at-home bleaching system," *Journal of Esthetic Dentistry*, Volume 11, Number 1, pp. 36-42, 1999.

Thitinanthapan, Waraporn, DDS, MS, "In vitro penetration of the pulp chamber by three brands of carbamide peroxide," *Journal of Esthetic Dentistry*, Volume 11, Number 5. p.259-263.

Wagner, Barbara J., "Whiter teeth, brighter smiles," *Access*, Special Supplemental issue, September-October 1999.

Chapter 7

ADA webpage: http.//www.ada.org

ADHA webpage: http.//www.adha.org

Allee, Verna, *The Knowledge Evolution: Expanding Organizational Intelligence* (Newton, MA: Butterworth-Heinemann) (1997)

Cantrell, J., Alabama dental hygiene program, informational letter, 1-4. (1999)

Darby, Michele, Walsh, Margaret M., *Dental Hygiene: Theory and Practice*, W.B. Saunders Company, Philadelphia. P.15-45 (1995)

Edvinsson, Leif, Malone, Michael S., *Intellectual Capital* (New York, NY: Harper-Collins Publishers, Inc.) (1997)

Eggert, D., "The systematic stripping away of dental hygiene's professionalism by organized dentistry took center stage in Topeka," *RDH*, 27-36 (1998)

Emerling, H., "The muffling of shout," *RDH*, 16-44 (1998)

Forsch, C., "Informational report on dental hygiene advisory committee," ADHA Nevada Constituent HOD Meeting 1998, 1-6.

Handy, Charles, *The Age of Uncertainty* (Boston, MA: Harvard Business School Press) (1990)

Jacobee, Albert G., "Humanities and the Culture of Work," Daniel Webster College, May/June 1998

Nonaka, Ikujiro, Takeuchi, Hirotaka, *The Knowledge Creating Company* (New York: Oxford Press) (1995)

Prusak, Laurence, ed., *Knowledge in Organizations* (Boston: Butterworth-Heinmann) (1997)

Roth, Sandra, R., *ProSpective, Volume One, Reclaiming the Passion of Dentistry*, ProSynery Press, Seattle Washington, p. 1-20. (1993)

Roth, Sandra, R. *ProSpective, Volume Two, Defining the Mission of Dentistry*, ProSynery Press, Seattle Washington p. 73-92 (1995)

Seltzer, Steven, "A futuristic view condex," *Dental Economics*, February, 1998

Stewart, Thomas A., *Intellectual Capital* (New York: Doubleday) (1997)

INDEX

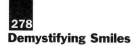

HERE'S WHAT CUSTOMERS ARE SAYING ABOUT SHOPPING ONLINE AT WWW.PENNWELL-STORE.COM:

"The service was great; I had my order within a few days — when all other stores didn't have it in stock."
— Scott R., Accokeek, MD

"I was very pleased with the service. Excellent response to my e-mail inquiring about my order status. I will be ordering from PennWell again in the near future."
— Chester G., Wilmington, DE

"I couldn't find a couple of items, I left an email, and they shipped the items as well. The online store is excellent and has my highest regards and approval."
— Scott E., Ilion, NY

"Being that I haven't ordered online at all in the past, the only basis I had for the quality and speed of service was the feedback from friends and relatives. PennWell has certainly made my first online experience a pleasant one…"
— Hercules R., Westminster, CA

"Already received the order and the invoice — it was quite user-friendly. Will definitely order again online. Thank you!"
— Brenda P., Denver, CO

What are you waiting for? Shop online today at
www.pennwell-store.com!

Don't forget to sign up for our e-newsletter to keep up with our latest titles and offers!

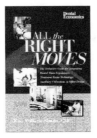
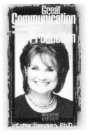
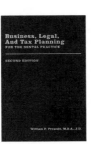
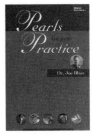